UNREADABLE TRAFFIC
EMS II

SEMON STROBOS

Copyright © 2014 Semon Strobos

All rights reserved.

ISBN:1502906503
ISBN-13:9781502906502

Unreadable traffic is 'medic' for garbled radio transmission.

Useful Abbreviations:

Board or backboard: flat surf board or plank like object to which trauma victims are strapped to protect the spine from further injury
BP: blood pressure
COPD: chronic obstructive pulmonary disease
C-collar: cervical collar placed around the neck after trauma to stabilize possible spinal cord injuries or cervical vertebral fractures until definitive care.
CHF: congestive heart failure
DNR: do not resuscitate
D-stick: blood sugar obtained by accucheck device. 60-120 is normal
Hot transport, formerly code 3, now priority 1: transport to a hospital using lights and sirens. As long as 'due regard' for safety is exercised, the only traffic laws which need to be obeyed are school zones and railroad crossing lights
IV: intravenous catheter
MOI: mode of injury, what caused the trauma, like high speed head-on collision
NS: normal saline, the IV fluid carried on ambulances for rehydration
R/O: rule out
Vent: artificial ventilator

CONTENTS

1	GSW, head x 3	1
2	Vocabulary	28
3	My morphine problem	29
4	When you gotta go	42
5	Randy Boudreaux	44
6	Harriet Houdini	50
7	The Super S crowd	57
8	Psych patients: the white slave trade	71
9	A dangerous profession	79
10	Hazing	115
11	The woman who ate her baby	117
12	The more complaints the better	127
13	Transported	129
14	Mr. Hutchins	154

1 GSW, HEAD, X 3

A GSW is a gunshot wound. We see quite a few. I had three to the head, and all three were walky-talkies, oddly enough. (Walky-talky being a trauma patient who is found able to walk and talk.) There is a moral, which I'll get to, but the stories first.

We took a call after lunch on a sunny day for a GSW at an address on I 35. We rolled up to a funky storefront, down a cantilevered caliche driveway. A pre-fab building with a built-on, pine lumber porch and stairs. I never found out what it sold, nor did I care. The proprietor, a middle aged woman, had been robbed and shot. She had been hit twice, once in the right humerus, which was obviously fractured—deformed and swollen--and once in the right occipital region of her head, right behind the ear.

Pudgy as a baby, but flabbier. Hair dyed orange. She was terrified. I was a little terrified myself, but I knew what to do. I had done it before. So the fear was just a deep background noise I was too busy to listen to. As focused as playing basketball, but this was no game.

The similarities with basketball are: that intense but wide open focus, the Zen-like slowing. Taking care of the ball, or if you're not the ball handler, then whatever is your job. Having the goal in mind at all times. Improvising a way to it. The teamwork. The main difference is that your Opponent is inhuman. Resourceful, but impersonal. More malign and more powerful, but not paying attention to you specifically.

I didn't like her. Fat, flabby, ugly hair, stupid. All that made absolutely no difference, of course, but I mention it to show how many things you are aware of all at once.

In *Earn Money Sleeping*, my first EMS book, I already described what going on scene is like for us. The acronym ABCD covers what we look for first in a patient, though even before we get to her we have checked out the scene on the way in. Airway, Breathing, Circulation, Diesel (transport).

She was being assisted by first responders, and she was answering my questions, though faintly. So her airway and breathing were intact, and the rapid trauma exam discovered just the two wounds described above. Circulation was thus provisionally OK until we could get a cardiac monitor on her and look deeper. As for mental status, she did seem confused, but just the shock and pain could account for that. No gross abnormalities neurologically, and we obviously did not attempt a neurological exam on spot. Instead we back-boarded and cervical-collared her as fast as possible, loaded, and set off down the highway to Wilford Hall Medical center. Big Willie.

"This is a load and go," one of the firemen said excitedly. No shit.

Every GSW or stab wound to the torso, head or neck gets boarded and c-collared, and transported to a level one trauma center. The reason is that the bullet will often impinge on the spine. I don't know how many patients I've dealt with over the years who had spinal cord injuries from gunshot wounds. Paraplegics, quadriplegics, a 15 year old girl on a vent because an errant bullet caught her high in the cervical spine, a 26 year old women, once very lively and attractive--she liked you to see hot pictures of what she used to look like, and to show you funny smut on her computer--who had

had some kind of fight with a boyfriend. A life of passion. She was still on fire. High maintenance from birth. He had taken out a gun for some histrionic reason. It went off. Perhaps he's in prison, or maybe not, but she didn't even blame him for it. She said he hadn't intended to shoot her. She was a DNR, though, and had become even more difficult to handle than when she was a princess. Lived alone with electronic help, even though she could only move parts of her hands and arms, barely enough to run a computer. Wouldn't go to a nursing home. Really a remarkable woman. Had I met her in my younger years, when she was walking, I would have been smitten. Everyone is attracted to some things which his common sense should warn him away from.

A medic got fired once because he brought a stabbing to a lower level hospital. I really believe it wasn't his fault. The stab wound was in the shoulder, which he took as an extremity. No arterial bleeding; pulse motor sensation intact. But it turned out that the stab went through the shoulder all the way into the chest. By the time the emergency room found that out, and med-com'ed the patient via a second ambulance to a trauma one hospital, the patient died.

Our lady with the GSW made it to Big Willie just fine, IV, monitor and everything in place by the time I got there. Staff was pleased to see her. They were training for Iraq, and don't get enough battle injuries to work with.

We were back at the station a couple hours later when we got another call for a GSW. This time it was a Hispanic male, 36, originating in a big truck stop, again on I35, though several miles north, into San Antonio. He was seated on a little metal chair, one of those ones with a red vinyl cushion attached. GSW to the right calf. It was not bleeding much, pms intact again, and no deformity. What I believe they call a flesh wound on TV.

His story was that he had been driving north on I35, had somehow shot himself, either causing a one vehicle accident, or shot himself because he had the accident. Years later I was telling this story to my then partner, in front of another non-emergent patient, and the patient said, "Oh yeah, that can happen. I shot myself in the finger once, and my dad shot himself in the foot." He and his dad seemed to think this was just one of those things that happen from time to time, like fender benders or tripping on a curb. Like another patient we had, a guy we transported because he was having difficulty walking. When he was a young man, he had been driving back from a hunting trip, with a 16 year old boy in the truck bed, when the kid dropped his hunting rifle. In attempting to grab it, he had fired it, sending a bullet through this patient's spine. He recovered and could walk for decades, but once he got older, more arthritic, the old injury put him in a wheel chair.

Anyway, our GSW patient had left his car behind and walked about ¾ of a mile to this truck stop, where one of the clerks had called 911 for him. We took him to a hospital, but this really WAS an extremity injury, and a mild one at that, so non-emergent. I did elect to take him to a trauma center though, since there was also the MVA to consider. I did not backboard or c collar him, as he had walked almost a mile already, and a thorough trauma exam turned up nothing but the calf wound.

The receiving RN said I should have boarded him, "If only for your own safety," i.e. to cover my ass. CYA. I really couldn't see it though. Sure, a majority of neck fractures present ambulatory, but they don't walk a mile and have no symptoms.

We got back to the station, and were contemplating making dinner while we talked about this. I made salad and spaghetti a lot that year. We could get the ingredients at the local supermarket, while listening to our radio for a call, and then later prepare them. Unlike fire crews, medics don't share food or cook much, but Cliff and I used to. I used angel hair pasta because it cooks in 3 minutes. I'd cock my head at the radio, hear no call coming, and drop it into the boiling water. We have to respond within two minutes, so I had only a minute of vulnerability, wherein dinner would be ruined. If I got past that minute mark, I could have Cliff get the truck started and call us in route, drain the pasta after its 3 minutes, and eat it in route to the call.

For Cliff, diabetic, the process was more complicated. He couldn't eat until after his insulin shot, so the fact that I was eating while he had to drive really made no difference to him. Besides, I always got him to drive, except when I was taking him back to base after dropping off one of his basic patients at a hospital. He was so much better at it than I was. An ex-cop.

So quite a number of times I was shoveling angel hair into my face while Cliff was riding the governor at 93 mph down one of our local roads to our call. It took at least 5 minutes usually and I could get the whole dish down in 4. Walk in wiping red sauce off my face. With indifferent success. It could have been blood, right?

I did drink a patient's blood once, but not on purpose. After I started an IV, I pulled off my glove and noticed a little skin abrasion on a knuckle. I reflexively put the knuckle to my mouth and licked the blood off, only to find there was no skin tear under it. But there was a tear on the knuckle of the glove.

We'd make the sauce too, but that could be turned off at any time. Even used red wine for it. I had to hide the bottle, since we aren't allowed to have any alcohol anywhere on the premises. The alcohol in the red wine cooks off, of course, so I wasn't actually imbibing any, but even the empty bottle would have got us canned. We like to live dangerously. Doesn't compare to wrecking the truck. Plenty of medic jobs around.

Besides, I can't make spaghetti sauce without red wine. White, maybe.

A medic got fired once because she picked up a six pack while she was refueling to go off shift, and then stored it in the ambulance to take home with her. She didn't drink any, but still.

You weren't even allowed to be in a bar with your uniform on, even off duty. Once in a while I would meet friends or my family in a Mexican restaurant/bar after work. I'd take off my uniform shirt, unload my unmarked EMT pants of all their gear and eat in my T shirt.

One cargo pocket has gloves and tape; the other has EMT shears, a pen and my paramedic field guide with its drug dosages, med lists, and various other useful info; one shirt pocket has a cell phone, and a pen light for pupil responses; the other has my company's business cards and a pulse ox. Wallet in back pocket, pager on my belt, badge hanging on my epaulet, and stethoscope around my neck.

It either stays there or is in my ears. If you lay it down it will disappear. Even seemingly honest firemen, medics and nurses don't seem to be able to resist a good stethoscope, and mine is very good.

I lost my Littman on a scene: the woman we found half buried next to a wreck, if you remember that story from *Earn Money Sleeping*. The same week my cardiologist asked if I had ever listened to my mitral murmur. "I've never been able to hear it," I said. He placed the bell of his scope on just the right spot, and put his ear pieces in my ears. It was like being inside my own heart. The murmur whistled like a steam kettle. So when I lost the Littman, I found a two horned, cheaper version of his three horned rhino model on-line and ordered it.

So I can hear blood pressures in a moving truck, at least sometimes, though I still used to have to take just systolic pressures to palp mostly, until we got cardiac monitors with automatic blood pressure cuffs. That saved a lot of time. And I can hear adventitious lung sounds even on noisy scenes.

Palp means you palpate a pulse with your finger, and then pump up the blood pressure cuff until the pulse disappears. That gives you the systolic pressure. The diastolic can only be heard with a stethoscope, but if you can't hear well, like in a moving ambulance with the siren on, the systolic is enough. You're not diagnosing hypertension in those circumstances. All EMS people know how to do this, but occasionally you will run into a nurse you're reporting to who is dumbfounded. Not an ER nurse of course. There are many differences between in-hospital and pre-hospital.

As we were sitting down to dinner, some things about this call struck us as increasingly odd. Not that everything isn't odd. The guy must have been very freaked out to both shoot himself and wreck. Then, instead of calling 911 from where he was, he walked a mile to the convenience store. Plus, he seemed edgy and nervous, a little off.

"You know," I said, "I think maybe we found our shooter. He's about the right age and ethnicity, he's a few miles up the road from where the shooting took place, a straight shot."

"In fact," Cliff said, "maybe he shot himself on scene. Two bullets in his victim, and one in his own leg."

"He could have some stolen stuff in his car, which is why he didn't want any cops swarming around it."

"Or he could be worried someone got a glimpse of his escape, and reported the make and model or even plate."

Cliff knows a lot of cops from his time in the service, and because he made even more of a point of making friends with them than the rest of us--besides he was a really gregarious guy—so he called Bexar County Sheriff's dispatch, which is different from ours, and which he has on his speed dial. He found the detective assigned to the case and discussed our suspicions with him. We still had our patient's name and info on our run form. We're not really supposed to give it out, but no one was recording the call. Seemed like a public service. Anyway, any gun shot in an ER gets reported to law enforcement, so the detective could have looked it up himself.

We never heard the conclusion of that story, but then we never do, so that was nothing new. We got involved in other stuff.

My second GSW to the head was a Mexican mafia gang hit. They had shot this guy in the base of the skull right where the spine attaches. This is their spot. Then they dumped what they thought was the body by the side of a county road in a farming area south of us, at a moderately busy intersection. They like to make a statement.

Normally that entry wound location would be lethal, but this time the bullet did not go straight in. It caromed around the interior of the skull, as will often happen with head shots, without causing a lot of damage. He was just dirty and scared. The ER doc later did a pretty thorough neuro exam and all he could find was some cranial nerve damage. And that was about it until the MRI and the neurologist had their say.

We don't get to see neurologists often. Very rewarding. That same week, we responded to a 40 y/o woman who awoke from sleep to find she was paralyzed on one side. Unclear if it was a short nap or after she got up in the morning. A poor historian, as we will see a bit later here. It makes a big difference when the symptoms started. A pleasant colorful messy Hispanic home. Patient sitting in a hand carved chair, draped by a colorful rug--or listing to the left, actually. Took a history: diabetes, high cholesterol, little overweight, seizure disorder, low thyroid.

Then we hotfooted it to the ER, since even though we couldn't determine when the paralysis had begun, so she was not a candidate for clot-busting re-perfusion, still, that's the doc's call to make, not ours. New stroke symptoms is a hot call. Her blood sugar was OK, so that was not the problem. She also started recovering feeling and sensation in her left side in route, so it was looking like a TIA rather than a stroke. A Transient Ischemic Accident or Episode is just like a stroke, except it all goes away within 24 hours, usually sooner. It does mean you have a 50% chance of getting a real stroke within 5 years, and much more likely sooner than later.

I had time to listen to the neurologist work her up. He examined her carefully, looked at our history.

"When you have a seizure," he says, "what does it look like?"

"I get paralyzed all down one side."

Bingo.

Why she had not bothered to tell us would be a mystery if it didn't happen so often. Patients like to make you look stupid. All the same, the neurologist had spotted the seizure history and asked the right question. We had not.

I once had a migraine patient who was completely unresponsive, Glasgow 3, though with good color and vitals (that turned out to be her type of migraine), but I had never before heard of a seizure with hemiplegia. Just shows you that while you expect certain typical symptoms, and do exams for them, still, since it's in the brain, a seizure or stroke can be anything. Attacks of rage.

Back to our Mexican mafia victim. He was knocked cold, but then woke up an undetermined amount of time later. He flagged down a passerby, who called us.

There was nothing else eventful about this call. C-collar, back board, rapid trauma exam, hot transport, IV in route, call it in, check interventions and re-examine, give report when I got there. It was more interesting for the docs doing the exam than for me.

Number three was at a military retirement community in our covered area. When we got there, a transport service ambulance was already here, in front of one of the neat, well-kept bungalows in the independent living area. Beautiful green lawns. That ambulance service covers that retirement community by contract, but in a case this severe, the facility wisely also called 911.

The medic, an Intermediate, came out to greet us excitedly. "GSW to the head!" she said. I don't usually react much to news like that.

Something freezes and goes on hold in my head until I get a chance to see for myself.

We went in to find a slender 75 y/o male lying in his bed, half sitting up, again fully alert and oriented. In a moment of despondency, or one of a number of such moments, I don't know, he had taken a 9 millimeter pistol he owned-- apparently he had found it somewhere, since his wife didn't even know it was in the house— placed the muzzle between his eyes and pulled the trigger. He had a small wound just to the left of the bridge of his nose. No other injuries on rapid trauma exam.

I asked him the usual four questions, adding "how old are you?" which I have to report to the ER from the ambulance. He said, "Old enough to know better." I got the idea: he regretted, what? The whole thing? Making the attempt? Not succeeding? Having to report all this to a bunch of strangers? My impression was 1, 2 and 4.

Again, back board, c-collar, platinum ten minutes and out, with his meds collected by Cliff in his spare time. Wilford Hall again.

"This is (name of ambulance service) 203, coming in priority one, with a 73 y/o male, found at home, GSW to the head, entrance wound bridge of nose, no exit found, no other trauma found, minimal bleeding, alert, GCS 15, warm pink and dry, 154 over 85, 78, 16, 97% on room air. NSR. 18 gage in left AC NS TKO, c-collar and fully back-boarded, ETA 10. I have a history and meds on board. O2 via nasal cannula at 2 liters. Anything else you need to know?" Usually they miss something, or I have, and they want to know more, but I'm really busy and don't have much time, so while I'm calm and polite--low, even and contained voice, like I have all the time in the world--I'm impatient to get to all the stuff I haven't had time for yet. A more complete trauma exam, looking at my interventions, the history so I can report it accurately, the meds, allergies, second cardiac monitor reading if I have time, second set of vitals, work on my run form if I have any time left over, check the IV I did in route in a moving truck.

    Let me translate: Priority one is lights and sirens, as fast as is safe. GCS is his Glasgow Coma Score. His vitals were: blood pressure 154/85, 78 heart rate, 16 respirations per minute, pulse oximetry 98% oxygen saturation in his blood on room air. NSR, normal sinus rhythm on the monitor. I had an 18 gauge IV catheter, running normal saline, in his left elbow pit, set at To Keep

Open, just enough drip so the line stays patent to use, no fluid if I have no suspicion of low blood pressure problems. He has a cervical collar around his neck and is strapped to a backboard against possible spinal trauma.

What you have to do, and report, is a little different for each type of call, and in every call there's a priority list, things you must get done like taking vitals, or backboard and c-collar for major trauma, and then a descending list of other things you would like to do, depending on how much time you have and how rapidly things fall into place.

There was period in EMS history when crews did everything on scene, but they stopped this as soon as they discovered that they were bringing in beautifully packaged corpses, and that the old 'throw them in the back of the hearse and roar to the ER' actually had produced better statistics.

Thus they discovered the golden hour, the maximum period before a trauma victim crashes, and derived from it the platinum ten minutes you're supposed to be on scene before transport. Which, as experienced medics say, Ain't gonna happen. You're doing good to get out in 15 or even 20, depending on the problems you find.

The doc asked my GSW patient if he had just received some bad news in the way of medical diagnoses, a common precipitating factor. Older people commit suicide oftener than younger people, and not as many adolescents do as people think.

The intermediate medic on scene was an odd bird. She has been described as looking like a 14 year old boy, as in "I didn't know we were hiring 14 year old boys now," except for bad teeth, and had been fired from my 911 service for attempting to make off with a couple fistfuls of Phenergan. It's not a controlled substance in Supply, so she had free access to it. I'm not naive about drug abuse, but I had never heard of anyone abusing Phenergan before. For nausea, it makes you really sleepy, which I guess is an altered metal state, if that's what you're after, and you aren't too particular.

Nevertheless, she was first medic on scene, so I let her run the call. I should have just taken it over, since I outranked her, but it didn't make much difference, and it was arguably the protocol, by courtesy. I ran the call anyway, but I did have to push her to give report over the phone in route and again at the ER. She didn't do a good job particularly, but Wilford Hall got the idea. We took her truck, with me and her in the back, and with my cardiac monitor along, and my drug box, just in case.

In a regular hospital, you help move the patient to their gurney, but in a level one trauma center you back off the patient, and let them move her. You start talking when you hit the door. You tell them everything you can until their ER crew starts their reports.

So what do we learn about guns and GSW's from these calls, and all the other ones not mentioned? Well, in the first place, this is not a venue for partisan politics. If anything is, unfortunately. I have many friends and medics who I work with who own guns. Most of them handle them responsibly. Not all. They are not about to give them up. Furthermore, the Supreme Court has ruled that the second amendment allows any adult citizen who has not been convicted of a felony and is not under a restraining order to own any number of guns. And it's their call to make. A significant and politically influential part of the citizenry is very attached to this particular right and exercises it with relish. So the right to bear arms is with us and will remain so for the foreseeable future.

The constitution is ambiguously phrased on the point, with that first, weird, dependent, defining clause—"*A well-regulated Militia being necessary*...the right to bear arms...shall not be infringed"--not because the writers were clumsy with language. The writers of our constitution were very good writers, actually. What they did, on purpose, is take one phrase from column A, and one from column B, and cobble the pro and con together to form a compromise. They did that a lot, when they could not reach agreement: not unlike the editors of the Bible in 400 BCE. Whose work they were familiar with. Look at the slavery text for another example.

So if you look up the Wikipedia article on gun rights, you'll find an excellent article. It describes how the controversy over whether individual citizens should have the right to bear arms, or whether only military groups should (as for example the state militias, which don't exist anymore), that this controversy has gone on from the very beginning. More than 200 years now. I ain't gonna touch it.

Limiting magazine sizes, banning explicitly-designed assault rifles, trying to prevent gun ownership by felons or domestic abusers or mental patients, even if successful, will have little effect on the 300 million guns already out there. If they have any effect at all, such laws will only influence mass shootings, which are just the tip of the iceberg. Most people who are shot are not shot in those situations. It will remain the case that more or less anyone can own more or less any kind of gun. The first thing a felon will steal when he breaks into a home or car is the gun which is so often to be found there. Privacy rules prevent us from registering mentally ill patients, and anyway almost all of them are harmless, in fact less likely to perpetrate violence than the rest of us. Plus, it's truly unclear, at least to me, that if guns become illegal—which isn't going to happen anyway—whether many people will still get them on the black market, as is the case with illegal drugs.

   So at this point owning a gun is kind of like driving a motorcycle, from the paramedic point of view. Yeah, you have perfect right to do it. And then that means, as a motorcyclist, you don't have to obey the laws about airbags, seatbelts, crumple zones, cage construction etc. which keep drivers of cars so safe. So it's your right, but it's not safe. Though not super dangerous, for most people, either. Even hunting, which hardly anyone wants to ban, has some serious risks attached, as does playing basketball or football, or skydiving. Not safe sports.

Horses are dangerous. You take an animal which weighs a ton, and is as nervous and as easily spooked as a 7 pound cat, and you decide to ride on its back, there is a very good chance that we are going to be picking you up at some point, or at least the pieces.

Also, if you want to protect your home, you want a shotgun. Maybe sawed-off to make it handier. Which is illegal, for reasons I'm not clear about. Handguns are fairly useless, as the above stories show, especially the small caliber ones. Consider a fairly typical outcome we had here locally, just recently. A drug dealer's client decided to rip him off. He made the rendezvous, and pulled out his gun. The drug dealer pulled out his own gun. The client was a better shot, or luckier, or first, because he got the dealer in the head. The dealer only managed to get his robber in the leg. However, the head shot turned out to be a graze, and the leg shot hit the femoral artery. The robber bled out before EMS could get there. And the dealer, relatively unscathed from the gunshot, is in prison for murder, because using a gun during the course of a felony does not qualify as self-defense, legally. Had he been selling a gun instead of marijuana, he could have successfully pled self-defense.

We have some highway ads here, for concealed weapon permit courses. They show a middle class mom--nice looking actress—sheltering her two kids—a boy and a girl, dressed like they're ready for church—with her left arm, while pointing her gun at an unseen intruder. Here's how that scenario happened. Mom hears person trying to break in front door. Instead of breaking in while they're gone, like a sensible burglar, he waited politely till they got home. Otherwise, if they walk in on him, he has the gun, not the homeowner, who left her other one in the car, naturally suspecting nothing. Anyway, hearing the burglar at the door, she yells, but he persists. She says, "Just give me a couple minutes, OK?" "No problem," he says. "Take your time." She combs the kids' hair, makes sure they have on the nice neat respectable clothing shown in the picture, rounds them up from wherever they are. They listen to her immediately and come right away. She doesn't put them in a closet or locked room. She holds them with her left hand, behind her, in the line of fire. She does this, apparently, so she can shoot with just one hand, as she has surely been taught to do by the concealed weapon class being advertised. Then she yells, "OK, you can break in now." Burglar says, "Coming in, ready or not!" Burglar is fortunately unarmed. Otherwise one or more kids and mom are likely to buy it in the ensuing gunfight. It's kind of a big gun, thus with a lot of kick, so, shooting it with one hand at an angle like that, she probably also shoots herself or a distant neighbor.

So if you have a restraining order out on someone and you don't trust that he will obey it, it may be the better of two bad alternatives to keep a gun around. A shelter or undisclosed location is clearly preferable to either, though. In a few cases like that having a gun may increase your safety. Statistically considered, though, for most people that's just not true. Having a gun makes it more rather than less likely you will be shot. Most of these are accidents, or result from moments of rage, or suicides in moments of despondency. Suicide is not usually a rational decision, under the meaning of the act, so depriving someone of the means makes a huge difference. Sure he can jump off a building or overdose on something instead, but the likelihood he will die drops substantially.

Kids will find guns if they are around, even if they are adequately secured. And lots of times, the guns aren't. Kids get to guns as easily as they get into forbidden web sites, or as they borrow the family car for a spin.

So the bottom line, for anyone with any common sense or talent for statistical reasoning, is that the more guns that are around, the more people get shot. This is the down side of your second amendment right to bear arms, just as there are costs to being able to own and drive your own motor vehicle, especially motorcycle, play the sports you want to play, fly your own plane, ride a horse, smoke, drink, eat junk food, drop out of school, or any number of other dangerous freedoms. And most of the above do have some consequences for others as well as yourself. But it remains true that most of the others primarily endanger only you.

From the point of view of a medic, these are the things that should be banned. Motor vehicles. Of course I can't see how the country could do without them, but surely motorcycles aren't necessary. Tobacco products. Horses. Dogs. Unhealthy foods. War. Guns for sure.

Of course, without all these things, I'd be out of a job. So I've heard medics say, keep on eating those burgers! Smoke those cigarettes! Drive drunk! Buy a motorcycle! Buy a gun, or better, lots of them! Job security for EMS!

So, obviously, I'm not drawing any political conclusions or being partisan. Guns aren't safe. The likelihood you'll protect yourself or someone else with one is miniscule, for most people, compared to the likelihood that something will go wrong. Out of the dozens of GSWs I've seen in my career, my calls and others', we've seen people shoot themselves or others by mistake, themselves or others by accident, but not once a case of someone shot by anyone other than a police officer because he was assaulting or robbing someone. I have read about some. It's so rare, it will make the newspaper. And of course the likelihood that nothing bad at all will happen if you own a gun is far greater, especially if you practice gun safety and act responsibly. So draw your own conclusions. It's a free country. And a really safe country too, despite all the dumb shit we do.

2 VOCABULARY

In Central Texas we get redneck and Spanglish among the languages we encounter. So here are some translations for medics:
Swole—edema.
All swole--stage 4 edema, as in "She's all swole."
Chakin--seizure.
Oogly chakin--grand mal seizure, as in "He was chakin. It was oogly."

3 MY MORPHINE PROBLEM

For my first six months as a paramedic I didn't use morphine (MSO4) at all. The luck of the draw, and the shifts I was getting. We use it for pain (not abdominal), for acute cardiac syndrome after the first three nitro's, and for congestive heart failure or end stage breathing problems under some circumstances. Severe pain, like a fractured hip. We can give it for kidney stones if we're pretty sure that's what the pain is (the patient has had them before for instance) but otherwise the thinking is that masking the abdominal pain makes it harder for the MD to diagnose the problem in the Emergency Department. Besides, opiates paralyze the bowel. That could be a good thing for some causes of abdominal pain. But really bad for others.

So I didn't know I was cursed.

The first time was a call for acute abdominal pain at a first aid station on a military base. The paramedic giving report there told me this patient had a strangulated inguinal hernia. Which clearly hurts a lot, given how my patient looked. I saw no reason to push him take off his neatly pressed uniform for an exam. Can't diagnose an inguinal hernia anyway. Painful waste of time. He was going to the emergency room in any case. Balls observed or unobserved. Take the paramedic's word.

He was a trim and well set up, impeccably uniformed 40 y/o male, carefully groomed, pale and drenched with sweat. It was clearly agony for him to scoot over from his gurney to our stretcher. I would have pulled him across on a draw sheet had I realized, but he did not like to be helped. Apparently he had waited as long as possible to report it too.

So any thought of him being drug seeking or faking it never entered out minds.

So we set off code three, lights and sirens, for Brooks Army Medical Center, the famous BAMC. He already had an IV line established by the on scene paramedic, and a first set of vitals.

I'd never seen anyone in that much pain at that point. But when I called it in to BAMC ED, the MD who answered the phone asked me why I was running hot. BAMC is unique in having MDs answer the EMS line, but it's partly because most of them are residents in training, so there are a lot of them, with not a lot to do most of the time.

I was nonplussed, but then I realized that I had presented the patient as perfectly stable medically and traumatically. Which he was, in the sense that he was in no imminent danger of loss of life or limb.

So I amended, "We can code 3 for severe pain."

"But don't you have any opiates on board?"

"I do, but I can't give them for abdominal pain. I could if you ordered it though."

"What do you have?"

"Morphine."

"OK, give him five milligrams IV."

"Yes, sir, five milligrams MSO4 IV."

"You can give him another five in ten minutes if necessary."

"Yes, sir, follow with five milligrams MSO4 PRN after blood pressure." MSO4 can tank your BP, but he was pretty hypertensive anyway, no surprise given his pain level.

Well, that helped a whole lot. In fact, after the second dose, he went to sleep. Vitals still stable though, so no problem. I thought.

When we got to the ED, we were met by the charge nurse, and the doc I had talked to. She appeared to be a very experienced, decisive and competent person. Kind of cute in fact.

And majorly pissed, as things turned out.

She stalked over after examining the patient and said,

"I don't see any inguinal hernia at all, much less a strangulated one."

"Well, that's what the sending facility said. I wouldn't know what one looked like anyway. Maybe it reduced spontaneously."

"Tchah! Besides, didn't you realize he was ETOH?" (Under the influence of alcohol. This would be a reason to be cautious about MSO4, since they work synergistically, especially on BP.) "How are we supposed to examine him when he's unconscious?"

"Uh, no, ma'am."

"He reeks!"

"Well, I'm sorry, but I don't have much of a sense of smell." This is true. I lost it, fortunately, early in my career. It was probably the second rectal bleed that knocked it out, or maybe the gangrene, or the wound with maggots in it. Or kneeling in the patient's vomit working a full arrest.

Then again it's supposed to be an early sign of Alzheimer's. This would have been her diagnosis.

"I didn't smell anything, either," the young doc said, sheepishly. He was having second thoughts about ordering morphine.

The nurse was by now too mad to talk.

"I'm not questioning your clinical judgment, ma'am," I said. "I'm sure you're right. Good observation!" This was not helping.

She snorted again and stalked off.

She was mad enough to call my On Duty Supervisor.

Rick Slaughter does not take any kind of crap from anyone. He was perfectly capable of tearing me another one for a minor infraction. But in this case he was pretty mild. He did note I had put the documentation in the wrong place on the form, but he's not persnickety. I was new. As he pointed out, if I had documented that the doc ordered the morphine, there was not much BAMC could complain about. I had reported everything accurately and documented all of it.

"You do know they can't examine him if he's gorked, though, don't you?"

"Yes sir."

It wasn't a week later that I used it the second time. This was an elderly lady who fell in her son's home. We found her supine with hip pain, a foreshortened right leg, and foot turnout on that side too. Classic hip fracture. She was in a lot of pain, so before we used the scoop stretcher to scoop her up onto our gurney, I knelt down, got IV access and gave her 4 mg of MSO4 IV.

The scoop is this ingenious contraption that splits in half so you can put one half on each side of the patient, and then slide it under her and latch it together again before using it to lift her. It's metal and sort of awkward but still the least manipulative way to move someone.

It does not work on beds. Gets tangled in the sheets.

The only problem I had was that the device we use to put the morphine vial into, in order to inject it, is, frankly, a pain in the ass. You have to take it apart, unscrew part of it, put it back together with the vial in it, screw it back together, screw in the plunger to the vial, twist the bottom to puncture the vial, and then depress its plunger to aspirate the vial and get to the good stuff. If you're not following this, neither was I.

You need to imagine this for a minute. You're on scene and, after struggling with a patient who is still seizing, even by the time you get to him, you finally have IV access and are ready to inject valium to stop the seizure. You know that people don't breathe when they are seizing and that this guy has been seizing for a while. The thrashing around he's doing requires a huge uptake of oxygen, so he's in imminent danger of anoxic brain damage, if not death. But the manufacturer or designer of this little device clearly feels that what you need at this point is a break. A little recreation. He surmises you will not have remembered to bring your Rubik's cube, or that little metal or wood puzzle you picked up at a tourist store, so he supplies the above described device.

A good thing too, because, left to your own devices, you would have injected meds without taking a restful break.

You may ask, why not practice with the thing before getting to this point? In the first place, you really can't, because the device can't really be practiced with, unless you have an unbroken sealed vial. Occasionally you may run across a vial that needs to be discarded because it's out of date, but in real life you can't just be squirting narcs into sinks without a lot of documentation. The authorities would like to know what happened to each mg.

Besides, in the second place, some things medics like to practice, and other things they get lazy about. Emergency medicine is an improvisational art.

I did get 4 mg of MSO4 into her, but I also lost 2 mg, leaving 4 still in the 10 mg vial.

Latterly, I tend to give 5 mg instead. 5 pus 5 equals 10, whereas 4 plus 4 leaves you with a useless 2 mg left over. And 4 mg is pretty puny for pain relief anyway.

As luck would have it, the exact same nurse was receiving at BAMC, where this lady went, owing to her being military eligible.

The RN had to sign for the wasted MSO4, which I did in her presence. Mostly nurses hardly pay attention when they do this, but in this case she was not only by temperament unusually conscientious, but already loaded for bear from the previous incident. So she flatly refused to sign for more than 4 mg, observing quite rightly that there was nothing like 6 mg still left in the vial, which was clearly less than half full.

So when I came in the next morning, there was Rick Slaughter again, with a little sponge on a handle, called a swab, which I was supposed to swish around in my mouth, and then put into a vial so he could test me for drugs. I had, namely, documented 4 mg used, and 4 wasted, which left 2 unaccounted for.

It seemed a little senseless to me.

"Rick," I said, "what could anyone do with 2 mg of morphine? You couldn't get a cat high with that, much less a 175 lb. man!"

"You could save it up, I guess."

"Well, but since I only used morphine twice this whole year, and the other vial was used entirely, how many years would it take me to collect enough to actually get off?"

"Shut up and suck on the sponge."

Well, I tested negative, no surprise, so that was the end of that.

But not the end of my morphine saga. I was obviously jinxed. I had a monkey on my back. Morphine just wouldn't let me alone. I couldn't kick the habit, seemingly.

We took a call in a rundown little house for a sick person. She was about 20, looked sick indeed, and was so woozy as to be altered mental. I got an IV going but, owing to her skinny little veins, had to use a 20 gage instead of my favorite 18, which is big enough to get in anything I want, but not so large as to be awkward. Meanwhile my partner got a D stick, a blood sugar, from the needle blood. As always.

It was 40. No wonder she was sick. In the old days, diabetics presented with high blood sugars, as their insufficient native insulin won't transport sugar out of the bloodstream. That's what diabetes is. Nowadays, though, everyone is under care, so diabetic crises are usually low blood sugar, owing either to the patient taking too much insulin, or taking the usual dose while neglecting to eat, or after throwing up their food, or over-exerting.

Well, the book says a 20 gage IV is too small for D50 infusion (IV dextrose), since D50 is thick and sticky, and is necrotic if it doesn't go into the vein cleanly. The patient was altered mental, if not too bad, so the protocol is, don't give her oral dextrose, in case she chokes on it. I decided to try to infuse D50 through the 20 gage anyway, carefully, since I wouldn't have put in the 20 in the first place if I had any confidence I could get a bigger needle in. Need to intervene NOW.

It went in just fine. So I learned something. If you're careful, you can use a 20 g for D50. Just make sure you have good flow, stable access, and watch it. Slow push. That's important to know, because diabetics often have terrible veins, hard to get big needles into. In fact I once saw a really great medic, a real artist with an IV needle, get in not only D50 and bicarb, but the entire full arrest pharmacopeia, through a 22 gage, which was all even she could get into that particular patient.

Then I made the family get the patient something to eat. D50 wears out quickly. She needed some carbs in her tummy. First they brought me a diet coke.

"But that's what she likes to drink."

"Yeah, but diet coke has no sugar. That's not going to help low blood sugar."

Then they discussed going to the store down the street for some tacos.

"Hey, this is an emergency, right? Don't you have anything she can eat in the house?"

"We have some Twinkies, but she doesn't like those."

"This isn't about her preferences in fast food, it's about keeping her alive. Come on, honey, eat the Twinkie. They can go get some tacos for later."

Very good, but, so, how is this a morphine story?

Well, when we got back to the station, we discovered that our drug box was missing. So we told dispatch and went back to the house, since we knew we had brought it in with us. It was odd it hadn't come out, because we look around for stuff when we leave, and so do the firemen who come in with us. It had been a confusing call, but not that confusing.

Sure, enough, they had the drug box. It was still locked too. We took it back out to the truck, unlocked it and checked the drugs.

Missing a morphine. The other morphine, the 2 valiums, the stupid device, everything else was there. But no second morphine. The lock looked fine. No evidence of any tampering, no scratches, no bent metal.

Also no second morphine. Still wasn't there.

So we report this to Dispatch. They send out a truck with another MSO4, which I sign for.

Also a cop. Another drug test, which we passed, again.

The cop's theory, clear from his line of questioning, was that the morphine never was in there, and I had neglected to check for it when I checked the truck upon coming on shift. But I was quite sure I had checked it. Cops, however, do not take anyone's word for anything, so that remained his opinion. He was gently trying to get me to admit I had forgotten to check, mentioning his own having failed to check on a loaded weapon once. That might be true, but I still distinctly remembered checking the drug box. Like every morning. You sign for it.

So this remained a mystery. Missing MSO4 from a seemingly untouched drug box.

Of course, when I told the story to the medic who relieved me in the morning, he didn't see it as a mystery.

"People on scene hid your drug box, so you would miss it clearing out. Then you came back, and a morphine was missing. Where's the mystery? They took it."

"Why did the lock look untampered?"

"I don't know. They picked it? It's not a very impressive lock."

"How come they only took one morphine and no valium?"

"You know you can never tell what junkies will do. Maybe they thought you wouldn't miss just one. Who knows? Junkies are totally unpredictable."

Well, I like that theory. But I have one of my own. Morpheus has it in for me. Need to sacrifice a chicken, a goat and a newt. Pray.

4 WHEN YOU GOTTA GO

At the new SAMMC ER, there are a lot of bathrooms, which is a good thing. It's a magnificent facility. Government at its best. But when you walk up to one, coming in from a run, after having given report, doing your Kegel exercises to keep from leaking into your uniform pants, the first thing you see is a sign which says, "Key on crash cart."

Actually, it turns out you can just walk in. The bathrooms are not locked. But at first I was imagining how I was going to get in. Find the crash cart, all bent over, squeezing legs together, and rummage among the cardiac meds, desperately looking for the key? Call a code blue?

The resuss team runs up with the crash cart, to see me standing there, no apparent distress.

"Where is the patient?" they yell. "In the bathroom?"

"No," I say, "actually, I just had to go to the bathroom, see, and…"

"You called a code blue because you needed to pee?"

"You don't understand. I REALLY had to go. It was, like, an emergency, you know?"

5 RANDY BOUDREAUX

Randy Boudreaux was a lot of fun to work with, and also a pain in the ass sometimes. Self-described as a Cajun redneck, Randy was an award winning fisherman. He had his schedule arranged so he could go fishing Friday, Saturday and Sunday. Mostly for catfish. He didn't hold with all that high falutin bass snobbery. He loved taking people with him, and would guarantee you a fish. Several. Fisherman say fishing without beer makes the day last a year, but Randy never made that mistake. Unfortunately, he got stopped by the cops after one trip and busted for DUI.

Though he got very little sympathy for this, it really wasn't as bad as it sounds. He was only driving down a little dirt road connecting his property with the lake where he'd been fishing. He got adjudication with community service. At first he was worried about having to clean up roadsides, but he found "they only make

Mexicans do that." Instead he worked in Goodwill for a while.

Another condition for his adjudication was he was not allowed to consort with known felons. "Well," he said, "the only felons I know are the ones they make me work with at Goodwill. And then, we transport some from jails and ER's, but I can't exactly say, 'I'm not going to transport you because you're a felon,' can I?"

He loved food, Cajun, Mexican, fish, and could cook really well. Age 32, he already had hypertension--they found it during his EMT class, when they were practicing taking blood pressures—so some of us were always trying to get him to quit smoking, lose some weight, or cut back on the beer, but it wasn't in his nature or culture. It would have been unmanly or too much trouble. At 6'4" he could carry a good-sized belly and still cut a fine figure.

At one point, we were in Methodist, in the ghetto, the room where they jam four or five patients at a time. Randy was standing next to the bed, having just transferred the patient. Irritated by the curtain, which hangs too close between the beds, he whipped around and started struggling with the curtain as though it had attacked him. Life around Randy was very much a slapstick world. "I'm sweating like a whore in church," he said after lugging a 350 pounder on a manual stretcher one hot Texas afternoon. You need some entertainment or comic relief from time to time. Need it.

But, on the other hand, was the day I told him to go a little easier on the turns during transports. He was a magnificently good driver, could "make a truck sit up and bark like a dog," but driving an ambulance is not the same as other forms of trucking. Gotta be very smooth. Randy resented the advice, given he was indeed a better, in fact much better, driver than I was. Better truck driver, not ambulance driver. So with the next patient he was really slinging me around. Problem was it was a patient with a spinal cord injury. Not funny.

Then, when I would try to nap while he was driving, he would turn up the volume on his favorite music station. Heavy metal. Not even I can sleep to loud heavy metal. He knew all the lyrics and played some himself.

New to EMS when I first rode with him, Randy never fully realized, in his heart, that transport medics generally don't share the food they bring with them on the truck in their cooler or lunch box, unlike folks who are taking a road trip together. Everyone brings his own. 911 medics, with a post to go to between calls, keep their food on post, but everyone else either hopes to get breaks, so they can stop to grab some fast food, or they hope to pick up some of the junk food set out for them in the hospital EMS rooms. Generally medics bring at least some food with them.

So Randy would act outraged when I wasn't sharing my lunch with him. And it's not like he was bringing me any of those fish dishes he boasted about to all and sundry. He would be driving and I would be cracking the lunch box. He would look over from the driver's seat, undisguisedly covetous. Once in a while I brought an avocado. This could cause a real mental crisis. I prefer eating them as guacamole or with some cottage cheese or hot sauce or picante in the scoop, but, that not being an option on the truck, I would sometimes just peel one and eat it with a spoon.

"I LOVE avocadoes," Randy would say, eyes wide with outrage.

"Well," I would say, "they sell them in HEB."

Once I actually had a couple bon bons along, though I rarely brought candy or sweets. Not that I didn't raid the candy dish at every doctor's office.

"BON BONS!" Randy cried out, beside himself.

He felt he was entitled to a full half hour between "destination" and "clear." Most services consider that a max, for when there are problems, but to him it was the standard of care. After all, he couldn't work on the run form during transport because he was too busy chatting with the patient, trading recipes, fishing stories, family anecdotes. This is not necessarily a bad thing. You like to reassure the patients and keep up good relations with them. But then he needed that time at destinations to finish the run form. After that, he also needed to smoke a cigarette, which obviously wasn't going to happen in the truck or at the facilities.

Periodically he would get dinged for behavioral issues, which never fazed him. Once he got suspended for two days for running hot down I-35 with his lights on but no siren. "It was giving me a headache," he explained, unrepentant. In his defense, that service didn't like you to run harder than 80 mph, which was where they set the governor, so in effect, you were being passed by normal traffic. We found it embarrassing.

The boss, who had some country genes herself, loved Randy, but there were limits. He complained ON THE RADIO about not getting a break to eat for his entire 12 hour shift, so he got called in for that too. Had he apologized that would have been the end of it—the boss was mostly focused on attitude—but Randy said, "You can't run 12 hours without a break for food," so he got fired.

You can, actually, but most people just squeeze in their own break on the way to a non-emergent call, or after dropping off a patient, before clearing. At worst, you can take turns driving and eating. "We make our own breaks," my own Field Training Officer told me.

Randy made his own job. He was working for another service within days. I saw him outside Methodist that same week. He patted his belly to indicate he hadn't taken my advice about losing weight, made smoking and drinking gestures, hopped into his truck and headed off for his next call.

6 HARRIET HOUDINI

Another Randy story. He hadn't been a Basic long when I first rode with him. Before, he had been loading boxes and crates for Walmart. So he could be kind of naïve. But very enthusiastic. EMS beat loading boxes all to hell. Especially for a guy with a bad disc from lifting.

We were transporting a profoundly demented patient. I can't remember anymore why she was in the truck, but it was Randy's call.

Only in her early 60's, she was unusual for a person with such profound dementia in that otherwise she was extremely healthy. She did not have other serious diseases; she was slender, muscular, lithe and extremely well-coordinated. She looked perfectly healthy in muscle tone, skin color, the way she moved and held herself, although she was only a Glasgow 10, where most dementia patients are 14 (just confused), or 13 or maybe 12.

Let's run it down. Glasgow Coma Score, 3 to 15. Made up from three categories. First, eye opening. Then Motor. Finally, Speech. First, she had spontaneous eye opening and was looking around everywhere, so that's 4. Perfect score. Two: She clearly did not follow or understand commands at all. It wasn't that she didn't want to; she had no idea what was going on. She just didn't have an inkling about what you were saying. But she did localize pain, that is, sensation, in fact extremely well (as you will see). So that's 5. Three: As far as speech goes, she had none whatsoever. She did not vocalize at all. Perhaps she could grunt or say something, but we never heard a peep. So that's 1. So 4 plus 5 plus 1 is 10. She clearly did not understand a word or gesture we made.

As I've said before (there's a whole chapter on it later, called "The Soul"), it's difficult for some people to grasp that another human being, who looks fairly normal, really cannot understand anything. They are sure that if you speak loudly and clearly to a foreigner he must be able to understand some English, given that the ability to speak is practically the same as being a human being, which they clearly are.

Harriet was a light skinned black lady with enormous luminous eyes. I would call them speaking eyes, except we didn't know what they were saying. In some ways it was harder to figure out what was going on in her head than a dog or cat's, if you are a person with a feel for animals.

We loaded her very carefully and gently, as always, to avoid scaring her, as most demented patients are very anxious, and no wonder, and kept talking to her about what we were doing, even though she didn't seem to understand a word. For someone who was not used to dealing with such situations, this would have seemed creepy and scary, or at least tricky, but for us it was almost boring. We did it almost every day. I always figure even if the patient can't understand, possibly the soothing voice will be reassuring. You tell demented people what you are doing, but you don't ask permission. What if they say No?

The legal doctrine is "implied consent." If someone can't consent to treatment because they are unconscious, or not alert and oriented, then you take legal responsibility for doing for them what you would want someone to do for you in the same circumstance. Really a kind of legal application of the golden rule, if you think about it.

We called her Harriet Houdini because she had an absolutely remarkable ability to escape from stretcher straps. The one fixed intention in her head was to untie herself and get off the stretcher. Made no difference the ambulance was moving and there was no place to go.

Randy tried everything. He put the sheet over the straps so she could not see or reach them. She burrowed under the sheets and had the buckles unsnapped in a trice.

He turned the buckles over so they were hard to get to and manipulate. It took her seconds to figure that out.

He tried to hold her hands gently. She wiggled free.

You cannot tie a patient down unless the patient is combative. It's a serious legal matter to restrain someone against their will. A felony, in fact. We can do it, but only under certain legal conditions, which she did not meet.

So Randy, at the end of his tether, tried to reason with her. I could hear him, in back, lecturing her at length about the necessity of keeping seatbelts on in a moving vehicle. He would have done a high school drivers' ed. class proud. He pulled out all the stops. Every possible persuasive device or argument was at his command.

"It's against the law to be in a moving vehicle with no seat belts on.... They're just seatbelts, we are just trying to keep you safe.... If we get in an accident you could be thrown against the wall and injured....Please, they don't hurt. See? It's just like a seatbelt in a car. You put on seatbelts in your car, don't you?"

Harriet stared at him blankly with those huge eyes, and unsnapped her seatbelts as fast as he could affix them.

Meanwhile, I was having a hard time driving, owing to laughing so hard. Trying to explain things to a person with dementia is a thankless and difficult task at best, but in this case it was beyond pointless. Harriet clearly had no idea what he was saying. Not a word. She had just about enough cunning to avoid his hands and wait till he was at one end of the stretcher so she could work at the other end. Her dexterity was remarkable. We have transported young, intelligent, combative patients who had nowhere near her ingenuity at unlocking seatbelts.

"All vehicles are equipped with restraints to keep you safe. They are required by law. What if a policeman stopped us? You wouldn't want to be arrested, would you?"

Randy was so earnestly intent on his task that not even heartless laughter coming from the front of the truck could distract him. He was maintaining rational argument even in the midst of struggling with all his manual ability.

I wasn't doing as well. I was trying to keep the ambulance going in a straight line while watching his struggles with her in the rearview. Tears were obscuring my vision.

We were flat out exhausted by the end of the trip. I was weak from laughter. For a good 40 minutes, Randy had been struggling, lecturing and dashing from head to foot of the stretcher in a moving ambulance too small for his 6 foot 4 frame.

"I'm sweating like a whore in church," he said when I opened the back.

Harriet was still fresh as a daisy. Of the eight straps we use, waist, legs, chest and shoulders, not a seatbelt or buckle was affixed to her person. Rodney had not given up either. But the quicker he had buckled them the quicker she unbuckled them.

Dementia is an awful disease to be sure. Harriet however, looked kind of happy. She was one of the few dementia patients I have seen who was not eaten up with anxiety, not subject to horrid fits of emotional lability or comorbid conditions. And it wasn't because she had succeeded in defeating Randy. That meant nothing to her. Nothing meant anything to her. For very long.

Except getting the seatbelts off. And as soon as they were off, she had already forgotten the whole incident.

Randy would have had more success playing basketball with Michael Jordan. At least Jordan would have said something, even if it was only, "You suck."

7 THE SUPER S CROWD

The first EMS job I had was as a volunteer for Jackson County Volunteer Ambulance Service. I had my Intermediate by then, but I was still in school working on Paramedic. Basic took 2 ½ months: Tuesday and Thursday evenings from 6 to 9 pm, plus all day Saturdays. Paramedic as a whole took about a year, same schedule, and cost only about 1200 dollars total in those days. In terms of cost/benefit, beat my other degrees all silly.

I went straight through the Paramedic program, though medics advise working at each level for a year before going on. But I started late in life and didn't have that much time, I figured if nurses and doctors can go straight through, so can medics, and besides I was interested in the medicine, not driving, which actually made me more nervous than performing medical interventions in the back of a moving truck. What if I got lost trying to drive an emergency patient to a hospital?

Now I could yell at my Basic for fucking up instead of my Paramedic yelling at me. Even better, as a Paramedic, I had really good Basics, mostly, so no one got yelled at.

Going straight through did cause me some problems. I still didn't know my way around the city, which was not good, though not as bad as if I had been a Basic driving a paramedic on an emergency call. Medicine, skills, radio traffic, emergency truck driving, documentation: it's finite, but hard to master all at once if you go straight through. I would forget to call "on scene." I held the microphone backwards for a while, with the receiver facing my palm instead of my mouth. Dispatch complained that my transmissions sounded muffled.

"Hey," I said, "Can I help it if I have a speech impediment! I try to enunciate." Then I figured it out.

I concentrated on the medicine and the skills and got them down for the most part. Following the protocols exactly, instead of using my judgment, was a problem, and documenting, sometimes. I learned that if someone had some pain in his chest area that didn't seem to be cardiac, I should put "intercostal pain" or "rib bruises" instead of "chest pain" on the run form, or I would get called in to explain why I hadn't followed the acute cardiac protocol.

Similarly, if someone had a bruise or laceration on his face that wasn't the result of severe blunt force, you had to put "facial abrasion" or "eye injury" rather than "head injury." Any head injury automatically gets a cervical collar and backboard, against spinal cord injuries, but someone who has cut himself shaving or bumped his head on a door doesn't count. Unless you're dumb enough to put "head injury" on your run form as chief complaint.

Jackson County was about an hour's drive from my house, and about 45 minutes from my school, so I would drive there after class, arrive about 7 pm, spend the night and the next day, until 7 pm, on shift. Many times I was the only one in the station, particularly at night.

Someone in my class told me Jackson County was looking for volunteers, so I applied, figuring I needed some experience. I soon found out that by working just one day a week, part time, for the service which covered Bexar County, I would get the same amount of emergency calls, and get paid too. Plus better training. But for several months I worked for Jackson County.

For years afterwards I kept their card next to my home phone. Every time someone called me asking for money, I would hit them up for contributions to Jackson County Volunteer Ambulance Service. That was a gas. The suppliant would say, "But I'm collecting money for The Police Whatever Fund. "

"Yeah," I would say. "I understand. I'm collecting for Jackson County Volunteer Ambulance Service!"

Or "but I'm calling from Washington for the National United Way, not just some county in Texas!"

"You mean you don't care about Texas?"

"Well, yes, of course I care about Texas but…"

"So, yeah, see, this is a rural county, but it has highways and farms, so people get injured and sick, you know, and we have to keep three trucks available, including one with 4 wheel drive, and we don't get enough calls to run the service off billing insurance. It's all volunteer, but we still need money for equipment, upkeep…"

Some of the supplicants would get really mad. Others would take me really seriously and promise to send a check to Jackson County Volunteer Ambulance Service forthwith.

In turn I would promise to support their organization, as soon as their check arrived. Which meant I never sent a dime to anyone, except for a couple organizations I had chosen to support without any phone solicitation.

Most of my time in the Jackson county seat, I spent studying my paramedic textbook or sleeping. We averaged about one call per 24 hour shift. I would answer the radio, put myself in route, and if no one else was there, I would coordinate with whoever was on call as to where I could pick them up, or if I should wait till they got to the station. During the day they had their one full time employee, who doubled as secretary and treasurer, but was an Intermediate who would go out on calls with me or whoever was available. They tried to take her off the clock while she was on a call, arguing that during that time she was a volunteer like everyone else, but she objected so vociferously that they relented.

We had some good calls, though not many. And they did do things their own way out there (despite having one volunteer who was the paramedic in charge of EMS services for the armed services), which is why I'm protecting them by changing their name and some details.

We took a diabetic emergency once, for example, to find, middle of the night, a comatose middle aged diabetic with a blood sugar in her socks. Took too much insulin or not enough food, whatever. Now, the protocol for this is IV access and IV D50, because someone who is severely altered mental may not be able to protect their own airway, and may aspirate oral glucose instead of swallowing it.

The other alternative is rapid transport to a hospital.

Neither of us on this call was protocoled to start an IV yet, though, and the hospital was not nearby. Plus the patient had elderly diabetic veins, anyway. Even for someone good at IVs, that would be a challenge. One I enjoyed on frequent occasions later in my career. Among the many IVs I missed, I was lucky enough never to fail on a diabetic emergency. So the RN volunteer I was with cajoled the patient, talking to her continuously, getting her to sip up, bit by bit, the oral glucose she was gently squeezing into her mouth.

Fixed.

We ran hot to someone who had been stung by a bee and was severely allergic. She was on a tractor in a field all the way down a dirt road. We scooped her up, asymptomatic, and I rattled their brains driving too fast back down the dirt road to the highway. Not too suave. I did tell the volunteer in the back how much epinephrine to use, though, which I did know how to do right.

They'd say, "OK, head the truck down to Peaville on Highway 16. Deborah will be in a blue Bonneville at the side of the road. Pick her up, she knows the address." So I would go roaring, lights and sirens, down highway 16, hoping I was going in the right direction. To this day, I have no idea what a Bonneville looks like, but I can tell blue from other colors, not being colorblind, fortunately. Not my favorite color anyway.

Once we got a call for an MVA at the Super S. My partner, the same nurse, knew where that was, so off we went.

When we pulled up at the Super S, we observed an old sedan--maybe it was a Bonneville--INSIDE the Super S, behind some smashed windows and doors, and the debris from a stack of pumpkins.

No patients though.

Well, they didn't want them in the Super S anymore, and it was too hot to stand outside, so they had sent them into the drugstore next door.

One elderly gentleman and three ladies, his relatives, who had been his passengers when he backed his sedan into the Super S.

They were all sitting on little chairs kindly supplied by the Walgreens employees.

They were not in any apparent distress. No visible injuries, and none on trauma exam either. No complaints, in fact.

Still, the driver clearly had to go to the hospital. The main question being, what had caused him to back his car into the Super S, through the double doors and the stack of pumpkins?

He claimed he had just hit reverse by mistake, instead of drive.

That did not cover it. He had kept his foot on reverse all the way up the sidewalk, through the first set of doors, across the foyer and the stack of pumpkins, and then through the second set of doors.

Still, no major trauma involved, in fact not much of any trauma, so he didn't need a c collar and backboard. We got him up on the stretcher, took vitals, did our exam etc. all per protocol.

Meanwhile we also examined the three ladies. No apparent distress or abnormal findings.

Except one lady, who had a blood pressure of 190 over 110. Pretty close to a hypertensive crisis, actually, though she said she felt fine.

Plus the other two ladies now had no means of transportation, and didn't want to be separated from their loved ones.

So we took the whole batch. The gentleman was on the stretcher, one lady was in the front passenger seat, one in the captain's chair in the back, and one on the bench next to one of us. We had to call all four of them in to the emergency room.

They were not real pleased to see us. We had just brought them in, seemingly, about half their weekly patient load. Plus no one had any injuries or symptoms of any kind. Lots of arduous paperwork for nothing. Even the lady with the high blood pressure was now normotensive.

"She's 143 over 85," the exasperated receiving nurse said. "You're calling that an emergency?"

"Well, not an *emergency*. We came in non-emergent."

"Whatever."

How did this happen? I took the blood pressure myself, so it was not operator error, not that a nurse like my partner would have gotten that wrong either. Being in an ambulance of itself would not drop her BP. The opposite, usually.

My theory was that she had forgotten to take her blood pressure medication, then, when she heard from us that her BP was really high, she had surreptitiously gone into her purse, taken out her pills, and swallowed them. She had felt pretty normal because this was not an infrequent omission. Should have seized her purse. I mean supposing she had pulled out her handgun instead?

So there we were, in the hospital EMS room, exiled from the treatment area by irritated nurses and doctors, working up run forms. Quite a lot of run forms. Four. That was about a week's work for us too.

So we're trying to remember which patient was which and which vitals went with which ones, who had the history of diabetes and who had the history of acid reflux, which set of pills went with which patient.

Quite a number of times later in my career I transported two patients, say from motor vehicle accidents, and it was always a chore to make sure the run forms were kept on the patient's bodies or someplace where I wouldn't get them mixed up. I'd have one patient on the pulse ox and the other on the blood pressure cuff. Two IVs running.

I once had to run hot with two critical patients because the backup truck was too far out. And that time I had a student on board who was not one of those military super medics just there to get a credential, but a totally clueless beginner who was completely in the way. I should have made him sit up in the passenger's seat where he wouldn't have been underfoot while I was calling in two patients, getting two IVs, follow-up exams, keeping the documentation in order and separate, switching the cardiac monitor from one to the other to get two readings etc., all in a flying truck.

That call was for a heroin addict who had crashed head on into a family car as he was speeding, going the wrong way on a highway while high. He was altered mental, head injury; and one of his victims, who I also transported, was one of the four family members, a boy who had been in the back seat of the family car with just a lap band seatbelt. He could not feel anything from the waist down, and had bruising on his abdomen, suspicious for internal injuries. It's easy to bruise tissue over bones, but bruises over the stomach require a lot of blunt force, like a lap-belt in a high speed head on. Tummy bruises are bad. Victim and perp lying next to each other, both boarded. 12 years old. Rest of his family in other trucks.

Still, the only real problem was at the trauma center, where I had to bring in the comatose driver while leaving the boy in charge of the triage nurse. I thought. She did not see it that way. Mentioned the incompetent student I had "left in charge" of the boy.

Who was up in trauma surgery in minutes, University being a wonderful hospital. I hope he can walk.

Lots of apologies and explanations required to keep my job on that one, but the nurse saw reason, or at least mercy, soon enough, so she never reported me. When I called it in, I should have requested help on arrival. Taking two critical patients was really unusual though. Only done in extreme circumstances.

My practice is, apologize often and copiously. Even if this one isn't your fault. Just remember all the times in your life you got away with other fuckups.

I learned this from my brother. He was apologizing to me for something once when I was mad at him back when we were in college. About half way through, though, I realized he didn't even know what it was I was mad about, or what he was apologizing for.

So anyway, back in Jackson county, there me and the nurse were in the EMS break room, trying to sort out the run forms and document everything appropriately, get the insurance info down so Jackson County would at least get paid for our comedy routine. What they call a clown truck, an ambulance with too many people in it.

We were stressed amateurs, and kind of exhausted, having been working in the Texas heat, trying to sort out all this stuff, none of which was what we had been taught to do, even for one, or at most two, patients at a time.

"Say," I said, "how do we even know these people were even involved in the accident at all?"

"What do you mean?"

"Well, suppose we just walked into the Walgreen's, grabbed four random old folks who happened to be sitting there, resting from shopping, and transported them?"

"Being old and forgetful, they kind of didn't object to anything a person in authority told them, so they just meekly went along?"

"I mean, they had no symptoms at all."

We both kind of collapsed into giddy laughter at this point, stress and inexperience pickling our brains temporarily.

Oh well. Another live saved. Four, actually.

If you feel inspired by our heroic service, please send your check to Jackson County Volunteer Ambulance Service, Pleasantville, Texas. See, it's an all-volunteer service, but....

8 PSYCH PATIENTS: THE WHITE SLAVE TRADE

Unfortunately, medics tend not to respect psych patients. It is of course very strange when a disease or condition presents primarily as bizarre behavior or speech. From time immemorial this has been considered to be in your mind, not your body. There is, however, no mind other than the one in your body, medically speaking.

It's unfortunate because a lot of an EMT's practice will be psych patients. Suicidal ideation, psychotic decompensation, drug abuse, cutting, eating disorders, these are our stock in trade.

Other than restraint or sedation, there's nothing much we can do about these conditions other than transport to the appropriate facility. Still, careful documentation and careful handling are in order.

I personally find these patients really interesting. Well, actually, the patients themselves tend to be aggravating and boring, after 15 minutes, but their conditions are interesting. One of the few things I didn't like about moving from EMT Basic to Paramedic was that the psych patients became my basic partner's calls rather than mine.

I remember my first one was a frail, dark haired 40 y/o lady who weighed maybe an anorexic 100 lbs. Her family called. We picked her up in the second worst neighborhood in San Antonio. Disheveled suburban houses, each inhabited by a different nightmare. She told us that she had stopped breathing that morning, and had died. She had succeeded in resuscitating herself, but was afraid it would happen again.

Her physical exam and history showed nothing remarkable, except a psych history and a red abrasion at the base of her throat, which she kept pressing. She told us that that was what she had to do to keep her airway open. There was nothing wrong with her airway or her breathing.

I was still an FTR then, a field training recruit, and riding under the supervision of Rick Slaughter, my FTO, field training officer. An extremely sardonic, clipped of speech, ex-football player and army medic who is one of the most competent people I have ever met, judgment, knowledge and skills.

When he got to be ODS later, On Duty Supervisor, he would answer the ODS line, called by him "the whine line,":

"ODS. Slaughter." Hard on the dentals and plosive.

"Wanna go to the hospital?" he'd say when he got on scene. "Hop onto the stretcher."

We asked our patient if there was anything else she needed to tell us.

"Well," she said, "I am worried that I will kill you."

Rick and I looked at each other. I'm 6'3" and an athlete and he, as stated, is a 220 lb. ex-football player. We had surreptitiously searched her for weapons during our exam, as always.

"We'll risk it," Rick said briskly. "Hop on the stretcher."

So my advice to medics with psych patients is this. As much as possible, treat them as normal people. Don't turn your back on them, but don't stare and look aggressive either. Mostly, they want to talk. Let them. Try to steer them away from obsessions, if it can be done unobtrusively. Ask about their kids or family. But don't insist. Mostly they want to express themselves. Their experience has been that other people are a whole lot less interested in them and their problems than they are, and they are grateful for a listener.

That's really about all you need to do. The command voice advocated by some textbooks is not a good idea in my experience. It may intimidate them, or it may make them attack you in self-defense. The medic I know who used it got his ass kicked twice despite being 6'5' and muscular. No one likes being bossed around, and psych patients do not take their disappointments in a retiring and tactful manner.

Mostly, they have no idea about how they are coming across. An extremely annoying, critical and insulting bipolar patient suffering a manic episode thinks she is just expressing what anyone would under the circumstances, and what anyone should want to know. If you don't take offence and take what they say at face value and with some sympathy, they often bloom. Sometimes you can even joke around with them, though that can go wrong, given how literal they are, and the fact that jokes are often an acceptable way of expressing hostility. Not acceptable to them though.

We had one bipolar lady who also had a touch of dementia and more than a touch of congestive heart failure. We were taking her back to her nursing home. A frequent flier. 65, poor health, obese, flabby, poor skin tone, disheveled grey hair tinted red in patches.

Part of the disease of bipolar disorder is noncompliance, unlike depression. They won't take their meds, have no insight and, instead of trying to make things better, seem to be bent on making life worse.

Pretty much everything we did was incompetent and wrong, according to her. Moving her to the stretcher was excessively painful. The sheet wasn't tucked in right. The stethoscope hurt her chest. There was no earthly reason to bang the stretcher against every available rock.

Besides, she didn't even want to go back to that nursing home. They weren't treating her right at all.

This creates several problems. A patient who is alert and oriented can't be taken against her will anywhere, unless she is 'emergency detention' for suicidal ideation or the like. And alert and oriented only means she can tell you what year it is, where she is, what her name is, and what is happening around her. A&O X 4.

Still and all, no one likes it if you won't take their patient where she is supposed to go. You have to enlist staff to do some gentle bullying to get her to agree to go where her doc needs her to go. Because if she is A&O, you can't force her.

The trick is getting them on the stretcher. They hate change, so once they're in route they usually settle down. Besides, then all you have to do is keep them on it. They're not doing the steering.

Fortunately, however, Brenda flunked her date test. We could force her, worst case.

Which still didn't mean she actually wanted to go, though. She was pretty consistent about that particular issue, even if her short term memory wasn't great otherwise.

And then, we don't like that particular nursing home very much either.

Combining some insistence with some distraction, we got her at least not to object too vigorously. The short term memory thing though meant it kept coming back up. Issues never get resolved for psych patients, or Republicans. Makes them aggravating.

So every couple minutes, she would say,

"Where are you taking me?"

"Excelsior Death Care."

"But I don't want to go there. I hate that place. They're mean to me."

"I wonder why.'

"What?"

"Nothing."

"What did you say?"

"You have to go. You need someone to take care of you. We're only trying to take care of you."

"Says who?"

"Your doctor."

"They suck. I'm not going."

Well, finally, I guess I had enough of this.

"Where are you taking me?"

"We're kidnapping you. We're going to sell you into the white slave trade."

She raised her head and stared. Her eyes got huge.

Oops, I thought.

But then she started laughing.

"Oh, they wouldn't want me."

"Sure they will. Fine looking redhead like you. We hope to get a lot of money for you."

She was delighted. In fact, she refused to let anyone else transport her.

"I want him in the back," she announced.

Unreadable Traffic

So even though I was a paramedic by then, I got to transport a psych patient again.

9 A DANGEROUS PROFESSION

Statistically, paramedicine is supposed to be dangerous, but I rarely felt at much risk. Bringing patients from facility to facility, as transport medics, wouldn't seem to be particularly hazardous. I think the statistics have to be broken down a lot to tell you anything. It probably depends a lot on where you work and what the standard operating procedures are there.

San Antonio is not a low crime locus, but we never responded for an assault or psych call or MVA without Sheriff's Officers clearing the scene for us first and remaining there until we left. I should have thanked them more often.

They are the ones who go onto a scene we have had to leave, a quiet underdeveloped rural neighborhood near midnight, because partying, noisy relatives of our high fever patient are getting drunk and aggressive, in their

Bandidos motorcycle gear, to the point we can't hear her lungs or get a manual blood pressure. Despite our pleas for quiet. "You just do your thing, man, and don't be getting in our space, understand?" We leave, and stage, and the cop, after stopping by us to hear the story, goes in all by himself. Soon, we troop back in to find apologetic Bandidos standing grouped in a corner. Even the beer cans still in their hands look more subdued.

Still, we do go into some gnarly spots on occasion, which I'll get to in minute, after dealing with driving.

Medics spend a lot of time driving, but not compared to truckers or taxi chauffeurs. Running hot presents some risks, but well trained medics who are following the rules can clear intersections, run against traffic or perform other maneuvers relatively safely. I was involved in three MVAs as a participant (rather than being called to take care of victims), not counting backing into poles, signs or into gates, which each happened once to me. That is, in the first two I was the driver, in the last I was a passenger. In fact I was asleep in the back of the ambulance, on a night shift, that time. Still had to suck on the sponge for the drug test though.

None of the three MVAs occurred while I was on my 911 truck.

The only one which was my fault was one day when I was transporting a psych patient to a psych facility. 281 and 1604 were under construction, to the point that you never knew what you would find there, even using the intersection daily. I was coming up on it from the west on 1604 and wanted to go straight, only to find myself in a 'turn only' lane heading North onto 281. I checked around really carefully, using all the mirrors, and went straight. "Out of nowhere" as all the ditzy MVA victims put it, appeared a funky sedan making the turn from the lane to my right. I whacked into his quarter panel, hardly more than a fender bender. We had to pull over, call dispatch, call the boss, and get it all straightened out, before proceeding with the patient. She was stable, otherwise we would have gone on without stopping.

I was so rattled that I actually drove through a stop sign a few miles further on. I saw it late and could have slammed on the brakes, but, as there was no traffic either way, I elected not to discombobulate my patient and the medic in the back. The patient's mom was next to me on the passenger seat though. She crossed herself. Must have thought she had drawn the most dangerous medic in town.

Another time we had come to a virtual halt crossing against the light over a four lane road, running hot. Traffic stopped in both directions. The second of the lanes to our left, the one nearer the center of the road, had no one stopped on it, though, and a pregnant woman, who was on her cell phone, somehow missed our lights and siren and all the other stopped traffic, and barreled through. I was in the passenger's seat so all I saw was my partner startle and flinch before we took her front bumper on our left front corner. Slammed our heavy ambulance over a good foot. No one was hurt, given how well motor vehicles are constructed these days, but the woman was transported by SAEMS, for being freaked out and pregnant, after getting her ticket for 'failure to yield to an emergency vehicle' from SAPD. The cops asked us if we had our lights and sirens on. That was all they needed to know.

Our boss wanted to know if we had come to a stop at the intersection. We had, and so stated. But the reason SAEMS had to transport the pregnant woman, instead of us, was that our ambulance was undriveable. We sat there for a while waiting for rescue and the wrecker, watching our back up truck speed by, heading to the call we had been responding to.

The third and last MVA actually made for a funny and illustrative story. We were transporting a demented patient to a long term care hospital for something. I was in the back. The patient kept complaining that his feet were on something hard, and hurt. They were. The oxygen tank strapped to the end of the stretcher. He was very tall. A stretcher isn't really made for anyone over 6 feet. I always imagined transporting David Robinson and having to leave the rear door open with his feet sticking out.

"My feet hurt."

Had it been a really long transport I might have had to figure out somewhere else to place the O2 tank, but, as it was, I just said,

"I'm sorry, sir; it's the oxygen tank. We'll be there in a few minutes and we'll get you in a comfortable bed. Stretchers aren't very comfy, are they?"

Of course, being as he had dementia, I was having to say this every few minutes.

"My feet hurt."

"I'm sorry, sir...."

When we got to the hospital, my partner, instead of going straight, then turning into the hospital parking lot, then over several speed bumps and around the dumpsters, elected instead to turn left onto the access road, cut across two lanes, and enter the hospital lot from the more convenient side, next to the ambulance entrance door.

Problem was, he had to scoot across two lanes rapidly without having another medic in the passenger seat to check traffic. He was using the mirrors. Generally he was a very good partner. He was most of the way through his nursing program and probably knew more medicine than I did.

This was not one of his best ideas though.

What I heard in the back was brakes squealing, honking, and then the ambulance swerving back to the left. He hit the cement divider, hard. I did not know that at the time. What I knew was that I was suddenly sitting on the jump bag, on the floor. After a few seconds, I figured out that I had slammed into the divider between the back and front. Hard, too.

It was so sudden and startling that I figured I must be injured. A rapid trauma exam, practiced on myself, however, revealed that I was not hurt at all. Generally, a medic who practices on himself has a fool for a patient, but I was just not hurt, period. At all.

So then I immediately thought of the patient. Crew safety comes first, so you could say I was following the protocol.

The patient was still neatly strapped to the stretcher and appeared to be all right.

"Sir," I said, "are you all right?"

"No," he said. Alarmingly.

I started checking him over more thoroughly. "What hurts, sir?

"My feet hurt."

"I'm sorry, sir…,"

What had happened was, by the time I had finished my own rapid trauma exam, and turned to him, he had entirely forgotten the whole accident. His feet were still pressed against the oxygen tank though, and this came to him as a new problem every few minutes, as he would have forgotten everything about what I said the last time he complained about it.

I checked him out a little anyway, but pretty cursorily. Unlike me, he had been neatly strapped in with five seatbelts, on a cushioned stretcher. I used to imagine a rollover, and finding a patient hanging from the new ceiling, still decorously strapped to the now upside down stretcher.

One side of the ambulance was pretty badly scored and bent and scratched, but, other than looking grungy, it drove perfectly fine, so unlike with the previous MVA, we just went on about our duties.

My boss had plenty to say to my partner but me she only asked if I was wearing my seatbelt.

"No, ma'am," I had to admit. I mean, I am a medic transporting a patient. Have to do exams, take care of patient problems, take vitals, deal with feet pushing against oxygen tanks etc. She felt I should be seat-belted at all times, though. "Sorry, ma'am."

Well, that takes care of 11 years of MVA's. Which are, I think, the most dangerous part of the job. We do hear about bad crashes, even helicopter crashes at times. They really are pretty rare though. Still, this is one of the problems, including excessive medical spending, that could be solved by better triage of patients, to be sure they really need ambulance transport. This has gotten substantially better lately, with Medicare requiring transporters to fill out forms that certify why patients need ambulance transport. Most people take them seriously. I do.

I did have a partner who had once been shot on scene. He had responded to a r/o arm fracture, and entered the house, to find that the woman patient did indeed have a fractured arm, but that it was fractured because her boyfriend fractured it. So this was an assault with injury, actually. She had neglected to state this as the cause of injury, or dispatch had neglected to ask. So no Sheriff's officer on scene to clear it first.

About this time, boyfriend comes crashing back through the front door. Not clear what was going on in his mind except we do surmise that he was angry. And armed. My partner threw his monitor through the plate glass window, dove through after it, tumbled and ran, but not before receiving a round or two in the abdomen. Required several surgeries, with impressive scars, and his digestion was never the same, but he survived.

As for me personally, I can only report two or three what I wouldn't even call near misses.

We transported a 16 year old kid back to his grandparents' house from the hospital. The reason he was in the hospital and being transported by ambulance is that he was majorly fucked up. Persons unknown, at least to SAPD if not to him, had on two separate occasions tried to cut his throat, and otherwise made several other nearly successful efforts to kill him. He was partially paralyzed. Multiple injuries.

My partner, streetwise, from the barrio himself, figured that the kid had run afoul of a local gang, and, clearly, one attempt had not satisfied them. He was at his grandparents' instead of his usual home because that venue had clearly not been safe. This was not an uncommon scenario.

So there we were, around midnight in the barrio, not a soul around, even the yellow streetlights too faint to show the ambient debris, which coexists with remarkable lush gardens, hand built decorations and artisanal structures. We were unloading, getting the patient settled and getting signatures. Up the curb, across the dirt yard on a broken sidewalk, up three or four wooden stairs, through a leaning screen door into a formerly porch-like ante room fixed up with a bed.

My partner then elected to clear and leave the scene as rapidly as possible. If the gang had gotten wind of where their erstwhile buddy was hiding out this time, and decided to come back and finish the job, we did not want to be anywhere nearby. We could always come back later to pick up the pieces, if any were left, after SAPD had secured the scene for us.

Similarly, when we picked up another assault victim off the street, from the defunct storefront where he was hiding, we hustled him out pretty quick too. My partner was scanning the lush live oaks and pecans in all directions. The operative theory is that an assailant may be on the way back to try again. Again, dispatch had not gotten all the necessary information—when do they ever?--and had not sent in PD in front of us.

The one other time I felt at some risk was when we responded to a call for a woman who had become paralyzed from the waist down, suddenly, per the caller. It was in the worst neighborhood in San Antonio, where the cops go in pairs and even the birds sing bass.

When we got to the disheveled house in question there was quite a crowd. Not only the extended family, but all the neighbors had turned out to see the fun. Most of them were drunk, or worse, but friendly. We crunched across the crushed beer cans covering the dirt front yard to the house. Residents apparently didn't even have the enterprise to collect and turn in their aluminum cans. We walked through a big front room and then down a narrow hallway, and then turned a tight corner, went through another tight, short corridor, to find our patient on her bed. She stated that she could not feel her legs or move them.

There was absolutely nothing wrong with her that we could find. She had no history. She was barely 40. She was healthy looking, alert, had good vitals, good blood sugar, everything you could want. Vigorous, great skin and hair. Strokes don't ever involve both legs, much less equally. Her legs also did not at all resemble paralyzed legs. The muscle tone, reflexes, color, tension, pulses, everything looked not just OK but strong and shapely.

"Did anything happen today? Did you eat anything that didn't agree with you? Hurt yourself?"

"No, we went swimming. The whole family was there. But there was an old woman there who kept looking at my legs!"

"Oh ho!" my Spanish partner said. "Ojo! I get it!" He was referring to the Spanish word for the evil eye.

It was a complete bitch to get her out of there. The stretcher had to stay in the living room, and we had to head and toe her, like a sack of potatoes, much to our and her discomfort, down the narrow hallways, and around the corners. Her drunk husband seemed not to be appreciative of our share of the discomfort involved.

When we got to the living room we deposited her on the stretcher. She seemed to believe that the more awkward and uncomfortable her posture made everything, the more earnest her condition.

"What's wrong with her?" he demanded belligerently. Tall, muscular dude with great hair. Now disheveled. His wife would have been attractive not long ago too. Fit. Clear glowing healthy café au lait skin. Especially for someone paralyzed. Cute couple.

"Nothing seems to be wrong that we can find," I said.

"Well, why are you taking her then? Where are you going? She can't walk, isn't that bad?"

"We're taking her to the hospital because you called us, sir. That's what you want, isn't it? That's what we do, we're an ambulance."

He took this as insolent and looked about ready to fight. Maybe it was a bit surly. I did feel at risk a bit here, but the crowd was not really on his side. Firemen and bystanders calmed him down.

'Sir," I said, "I'm just trying to help your wife. I'm trying to take care of her and take her to the hospital so they can figure out what's wrong. Isn't that what you want? I'm not a doctor."

He became very apologetic, in fact lachrymose. Requiring even more attention.

So that didn't make me feel all that much better. I wasn't going to pull my crew, leave the scene and get police officers involved, but I did intend to hustle out of there as quickly as possible. Drunks are labile. Sure I was his best friend and long lost soul-mate and hero right now, but two minutes from now he might be back in the aggrieved husband mode, defending his wife's honor.

We took her to South Central. It was busy and the receiving nurse was in an even worse mood than he usually is. This is a guy who is a terrific nurse. He knows a lot, he's totally involved in patient care, and his judgment and practice are impeccable. It's a treat to watch him sitting next to a patient, even after taking report, studying her, oblivious of everything, including your gaze, while he makes sure he's done everything he needs to do, and figured out everything he needs to figure out.

His bedside manner, however, sucks. His chunky body tends to bend forward aggressively, abetted by spiky hair sticking out in all directions. In fact he tends to be rude to everyone, medics included. I know him and he knows me so I can get him off his horse, but over time I have found him working in a lot of different ERs. I surmise it's his manner. A kindred soul, actually.

He assigned our patient to a chair by the triage room to wait for her PA exam, instead of to a bed to await the MD. We unloaded her there, awkward as ever. When we left she was balancing, chicken-like, half on the seat, half scraping onto the floor, holding herself up. Paralyzed legs *stiff*. A truly paraplegic person cannot sit in a chair, of course, but he was not buying it.

On occasion, we get truly dangerous psych patients. Much of the time you can just ask them if they are a danger to you, and they will answer honestly, or at least illustratively. Then you pull out and stage until PD has a chance to assess the situation. You can, if need be, transport with an officer in the back with you. Cops generally prefer to follow you in their own unit, not liking to leave it, but that won't always do. You have to twist their arm. Cop arms don't twist easy.

Once we picked up what I still think was a small gorilla at Santa Rosa Children's. That is, he was described to us in the paperwork as a 14 year old male, i.e. human, but he had that those completely flat broad cheekbones, primate eyes, weighed well over 200 lbs., and his knuckles dragged when he walked. Which he didn't do a lot of.

No one was in his cubicle/room with him, when we got to Santa Rosa. His grandma was nearby. She was totally intimidated by him, and warned us not to turn our backs on him. She obviously hadn't ever told him to do anything he did not want to do in many years, and with good reason. As a result of her common sense she was still able to walk and talk normally.

Not only were we not going to turn out back on him, we were not going in the room at all. Santa Rosa reasonably concurred that some sedation was in order.

Two cops showed up. Off duty, they were moonlighting as hospital security. I watched their operation with fascination.

They stood in the doorway and faced our patient. The gorilla picked up a chair to threaten them with. They both squared off at him and ordered him to put the chair down. Up to then they had been deliberately nonconfrontational, had in fact ignored the patient and not even made eye contact.

Gorilla put chair down.

Officer number one then entered the gorilla's room, once again ignoring him, and started picking up and straightening up chairs and other furn that had been displaced. He did indeed turn his back on the gorilla during this.

However, the other officer was still standing in the doorway facing the patient directly. I gathered he was in position to warn the first officer and intervene in the event of attack.

Pretty soon gorilla kind of loses track of officer number one, attending to the one in front of him facing him. The moment gorilla turns his back on officer number one, though, he turns, slams into the gorilla, grabs him around the chest and arms with both arms, and drops him onto the floor prone, falling onto him. Officer two leaps forward, grabs gorilla by the feet, which he bends up at the knees to immobilize him.

Gorilla pleads for mercy. He faintly resembles a 14 year old boy now.

Nurse runs in with syringe containing 2 of Haldol and 3 of Versed. Injects it into the back of the thigh thru the pants.

When I injected the same cocktail into a noncompliant epileptic kid who became violent post ictal, I had prissily rolled up his sleeve and put it into his bicep. That 21 y/o kid was a muscular athlete, standing on his bed, but we had the bed surrounded by a cop, four firemen and four medics, so our only concern was not to hurt him. Still, though it was not physically dangerous for us, it was eerie and scary in an emotional sense, troops in the middle of the night, an insane, terrified, lean jock glaring wildly from on high. A young fireman had moved directly in front of him, making full eye contact with dreamy eyes, shoulders relaxed and ready. The epileptic kid screamed in enraged terror.

Officers continue to sit on the boy. They let him up after he evinces submission, and help us tie him onto our stretcher. Gorilla then spits at my partner. Partner puts N3 mask on his face. Boy says "I can't breathe I can't breathe take it off."

He can breathe. He can even talk.

Partner says, "I'll take it off, but if you spit again, it goes back on, and then it stays on, no matter what you say. Understand?"

Partner does not perform said action until boy nods contritely.

By now the Haldol had kicked in so we had no further problem with the boy. He was never informed of the injection, given that this was known to upset him. We delivered him to a pediatric psych facility, which was quite familiar with him, followed by one of the officers, in his unit, who was never needed. He complained about my driving. Said I kept getting him stuck in the wrong lane. Because I wasn't sure how to get there. One of my first transports.

We had another one of these known troublemakers, who we were assigned to take from an ER to a sister hospital with a psych floor. When I peeked in his room, around the officers, I saw a 30 y/o well groomed middle sized but quite muscular guy wearing a clean check short sleeve shirt. His short blond—colorless--hair was neatly combed and lightly jelled into place. He appeared quite normal, though perhaps a bit vacant and mildly alarmed, but there was a faint air of menace palpable.

I was told by the charge nurse that he would be trouble and that "he fights." In that case, I suggested, perhaps some chemical restraint would be useful.

"Well, we have orders for some, but it never got here from the pharmacy."

"Maybe we should wait till it does get here." I knew they wanted their bed, but at present this was no emergency. It could become one.

"Are you refusing to transport the patient?"

"No," I said.

The nurse was a little agitated, overworked and under pressure, so she didn't follow the double negative. She called my boss, stating I was refusing to transport. Not at all, I told her, I just think he should get the Zyprexa they ordered, so no one gets hurt, patient or providers. Chemical restraint is far preferable to physical restraint.

My boss thought that sounded like an excellent idea, and even the nurse saw reason. I actually like her. She's a homey, plain kind of person, outspoken, not careful enough about getting out of her depth. She remembers you—well, of course she remembers me, after this—and is friendly when you run into her.

So two policemen, two nurses, two medics and bystander or two went into the patient's room to talk him into taking his meds.

At first he didn't seem inclined to cooperate. The nurse told him it would make him feel better. He considered this. He was really kind of an unusual psych patient. Well dressed and groomed, ordinary rather than bizarre in manner, and we were reasoning with him. He was considering his choices rationally. He was calm. Though the potential for an explosion was evident to everyone.

I kind of liked him too. I could sympathize with his position. No one likes to be forced to do something, not even children. Unfortunately we are constantly dependent on other people; powerful individuals and groups can fuck us over bad. You learn to play the angles, you can employ the Putney Swope maneuver of laying low, not attracting any attention. Some players even enjoy and excel at the politics, in the original sense.

But if it was a pity to have to force him into the loony bin, there wasn't much to be said against it. He had not only threatened violence against others but he had already acted on his threats. He could get out in a day or two merely by acting rationally. If that was not in his power, well, we didn't want him at large.

The officer said, "I really don't want to get hurt on the job. I've got a wife and kids. On the job injuries really mess things up for everyone for a long time. So instead of us tying you down by force, I suggest you cooperate." I was impressed. While playing weakling with his sob story, he had clearly implied, in a way this patient fully understood, that the end result, one way or another, was going to be the patient tied down on the stretcher, and that if someone was going to get hurt accomplishing this end, the most likely candidate was going to be him. This guy had dealt with cops before. He may have been delusional or under the influence of some variety of illusions, but they did not include the likelihood of him beating up on weak ineffectual cops.

Patient was crazy, but not stupid. He looked at the 6 of us and considered again who was most likely to get hurt. He took his med.

It was nowhere near enough Zyprexa, though. He was OK getting onto the stretcher, as per agreement, but as soon as we started applying the soft restraints, he started to struggle. A misunderstanding. He was imagining that if he cooperated now we would transport him unrestrained. Given his recent history, in fact, given the last five minutes of negotiation, that was not going to be the procedure in my truck. A moving vehicle with one medic next to him, rather than 6 personnel. So five of us held him down while I tied his feet, his legs, his hips, his chest, his upper arms, his elbows and his wrists, using knots I had learned in sailing class, designed to hold a bucking 6 ton craft in a force 4 gale.

He gave up, at least for the time being. My partner sat by him in the back and was talking quite reasonably to him. As I've said, psych patients are most alarmed by change. Once they are secure in the back, the tricky moment doesn't come until you unload.

Sure enough, we are trying to get him registered at the ER reception desk of the hospital, as Admit is closed, and he is struggling again. I ask the clerk to call security. She seems either to be half sleep or to imagine I want security in 15 or 20 minutes. "I mean, RIGHT NOW," I tell her. "In fact five minutes ago."

One slender security agent appears. This one is no off duty officer. I can tell because officers have to weigh at least 130 pounds and be 21 years old. They have streetwise, alert expressions—that cop look—and do not show fear. Certainly not of unarmed psych patients. They convey the impression that this is not the first time they have ever restrained someone.

The three of us manage to get our patient into the elevator to the third floor and then out right in front of the locked door leading to the ward. We ring the bell. At this point my partner has to remove the oxygen tank from the stretcher because the patient is kicking it loose. With only two of us holding him, the patient manages to get an arm free. He has somehow managed to evade my elbow restraint.

Let me put in a few tips here for anyone who is planning to kidnap someone or lawfully transport him in restraints. It is possible, in fact fairly easy, to tie someone up so they cannot move. They may lose the circulation to a hand or foot and have to have it amputated, or be choked to death, but they will not get free. Similarly, you can gag someone so that he cannot scream. But a person who cannot scream generally also cannot breathe. So if you don't care whether the person arrives one piece and alive the restraining process isn't difficult. Restraining someone safely, though, is quite another art. To do it right you need cuffs, leg irons, and some other illegal-for-civilian's equipment not normally carried on an ambulance. We do transport prisoners with a law enforcement officer in attendance, and they will not escape, cause any trouble or arrive in worse shape than they left: in cuffs, leg irons, multiple chains and locks.

    My partner comes back and the three of us are struggling with him. He's really strong. Later I realize that, while obstreperous, our patient is playing fair. He is not biting or butting. We in turn are doing our best not to hurt him. No one is punching.

    The locked door opens. A large black lady of mature age appears. Something strange happens to the atmosphere. All four of us immediately somehow feel like schoolboys who have been caught fighting by the principal, even though I am, actually, older than she is.

"John," she says in a loud no nonsense voice.

John freezes.

"John," she says. "I want you to come in here, sit in that chair and behave yourself. You know the rules here, and you know what happens when you act up."

John is mesmerized.

"Yes ma'am," he says.

We untie him. Actually, cut all the restraints off with our shears. John meekly steps off the stretcher, walks to the chair next to the vitals machine, and sits down.

"That's better," the lady says. "We're glad to see you again, as long as you behave."

"Yes, ma'am," John says.

So the command voice does work for some people. I can tell you with no shame that I did everything the lady wanted too. I would not have crossed her either. Though perhaps John had been brought to reason by some memory of events during his last visit.

The command voice has never worked for me though. I've described how I prefer to let the patients vent whatever they have on their minds, and how I try to be agreeable. Usually works. Whereas one of my mentors and field training officers preferred the command voice and came to grief with it. Despite being 6' 5", 200 pounds and muscular, he did not have the command presence of the nurse in the locked ward.

He arrived on a psych scene once to observe several police vehicles. He naturally assumed the scene had been cleared and was safe.

He entered the house and proceeded to the bathroom where he had heard noise. In the tub, taking a bath, was 30 y/o strongly built woman, who was clearly and obviously not in her right mind, judging by speech and behavior. When questions went unanswered and reasoning ditto, Jack tried the command voice. When that had no effect, he and his partner seized the patient and tried to maneuver her onto their stretcher. She screamed for help.

Her husband, who was also a police officer, appeared in the bathroom door. He observed two males struggling with his screaming naked wife. A melee ensued, two against two, with the police officers probably better trained and more experienced than the medics. Jack's partner did however manage to grab the patient's hand when she was attempting to insert a pencil in Jack's ear, using a vigorous stabbing motion which could have driven the pencil right thru the ear into Jack's brains. A large enough target at short range.

I have heard the tape of this call. Jack had the radio still attached to his hip and can be heard screaming for back up. Fortunately neither officer had his or her service revolver to hand, and at least the male component, of sane mind, eventually grasped the full picture.

Jack was on the injured list for two weeks though.

Still and all, though, in 11 years of practice, this is as near as I have come personally to being in danger. I think it sounds worse than it is, if you pick the near misses and other medic's overheard experiences. I have friends in Texas who are not medics and never deliberately got into harm's way but who nevertheless have been shot at or walked in on burglars, to say nothing of the military folks I know whose experiences have been immeasurably worse.

Actually the only time in 11 years I really felt I was in any imminent danger was when I was on a chest pain call with my all-time worst partner. I soon managed to get rid of her. Many people found her attractive, though not me, as she is not the kind of loon I go for. So I was able to trade her to another paramedic for two pounds of coffee. His wife worked in Starbucks.

We actually transported her once. Cliff and I got a call for an unconscious unknown and set off.

"Hey," I thought, "this is Mickie's neighborhood."

"Hey," I thought, this is Mickie's street."

"Hey," I thought, "this is Mickie's house."

"Hey," I thought, "that's Mickie's SUV," seeing the first responders clustered around it. I still didn't quite believe it.

"Hey," I thought, "it's Goldilocks, uh, Mickie."

She was "unresponsive." She looked fine, though, and I found that I felt not the least alarmed. My clinical instincts were not ringing any alarm bells. Sure enough, her vitals were fine, blood sugar fine, everything, color, tone perfectly normal. And she was talking to me. As I started the IV, I said, "Well, you won't have to clean up the blood this time, at least," which is something she used to complain about. She smiled, eyes still closed.

Paramedics have a reputation for being messy sticks. Another partner used to say, "Hey, Semon, what is it with all the blood back here? Bleeding the patient went out in the 19th century."

"Well," I said, quoting John McCain, "if this is an emergency, there's going to be blood in the floor."

I did transport Mickie code three to Wilford Hall though. I mean, supposedly she was unconscious.

The doc wasn't buying it either. "Conversion symptoms," he said. "This is your partner? Is she kind of a strange person?"

"Yes," I allowed.

Staff were all looking at me. They were not sure whether to be sympathetic, or suspect that I might not be working with a full deck myself. What kind of medic would have a partner like that?

"It must be weird to transport your own partner," one said.

"Yes," I said, "it is." I was in fact kind of speechless. So that response didn't give them enough to work with. They were inclined to be kind, but also not to get too close.

The chest pain call however was something else. When we got on scene we found a 40 y/o healthy looking Hispanic woman in a nice modest suburban home. She stated she was having chest pain. It was pretty clearly anxiety, however, given the patient's age, history and demeanor. Nevertheless, chest pain is chest pain, so I was soon in the back working through the acute cardiac algorithm, not going overboard with the nitroglycerin, though.

Mickie was god knows where, which is not where your partner is supposed to be.

Pretty soon, though, the rear door pops open, and Mickie shoves a 17 year old boy into the back of the ambulance. No one is supposed to be there except me, the patient, and maybe the mom of a Pedi patient, and even then only with my invitation.

"He's got a gun," Mickie says.

"WHAT?!" I said. What I meant was, then what the hell is he doing in the back of my truck?

Mickie disappears again before answering.

It turns out however that Mickie did not mean this young man, the patient's son, but another young male who was attempting to shoot this one. Now, it will be obvious to everyone else but Mickie that it is not the function of an emergency ambulance service to rescue people who are being shot at. An ambulance is far from bullet proof, and not only us, but the patient we are trying to take care of, are not either.

Mickie however by this time being gone again, I continued to work up my patient, that being my job and not having anything else useful to contribute. Making the patient's son get out was not going to accomplish anything, other than waving a red flag at his assailant, and further agitating my anxiety patient, who was not taking this well at all. By now, she WAS having a heart attack, in the metaphorical sense that is. Physical heart still stable, if stressed.

Then I hear Mickie hop into the driver's seat and take off. This represented an improvement in the situation, in my opinion. But the problem was that this subdivision had only one entrance, and the patient's house was right next to it. So we had to drive forward deeper into the small subdivision, just two parallel streets, linked at the ends, and then circle back to the entrance, driving by the afflicted house again, while never really being out of earshot or sight of our alleged shooter.

This was substantially worse than the time we were staging for a gunshot wound in a subdivision and heard over our radio that the shooter had exited the house and was at large somewhere in the subdivision. Or the time we were staged on a highway, a mile from the scene of a family disturbance, only to find out later that the perpetrator had been hiding under the same highway overpass where we were. We found out because the police came by, complaining that their dog didn't bite him. The other division's dog did bite, but theirs seemed disinclined, much to their chagrin. When we heard about the at large shooter in the subdivision I asked my partner if his bullet proof vest was big enough for two people. I had been making fun of it all day too so my partner answered "no" with discernable satisfaction.

Anyway, we made it out of our anxiety patient's subdivision without further incident. Acute cardiac calls require a lot of attention, so I was paying minimal attention to Mickie's chaos at the time.

Given certain lapses in her grip on reality, I never did find out for sure what the whole story had been. The shooter may have just had a pellet gun. I did not hear any shots. But who knows?

I did make a real murder scene with Mickie once, though. We got a call for a sick person. We were on the way, when I got a page saying to be careful because a child had made the call, and it was unclear to the dispatcher what was going on. The child had said someone was unconscious or dead or collapsed or some such. I did not communicate the page to Mickie, which became a bone of contention later. I didn't know what to make of it.

When we got there, we turned into a complex of run-down buildings off I 35. There were two fire trucks in front of us and a police car behind us so I didn't feel the scene was insecure. I let the officer park and access the scene before I did. He did not seem alarmed either.

We walked into a pre fab rickety structure through a broken screen door. There was a huge mess inside. On a filthy bed was a 25 y/o male, lying on his side among some dirty sheets. He was pale. He had 21 tiny blue spots scattered around his body, which we recognized as entrance wounds for a small caliber gun. We did not count them. I learned this from the prosecutor who interviewed me later. I put a monitor on the victim for the form of the thing, but he was cold and stiff and had dependent lividity underneath, so I just took a cardiac reading for the run form. Asystole in two leads.

This scene now belonged to law enforcement, not to us.

We walked out. Two women were sobbing and clinging to each other near the door. I did not like them. I did not like their tears. I did not like their environment. There was nothing at all I saw that I liked.

Mickie however was soon over there hugging and consoling them, while I proceeded to my ambulance. If she got in trouble, the police, all over the place, could take care of her.

She told me one was the deceased's sister and the other was his common law wife.

Which of course made them prime suspects. And indeed it soon turned out that the perp was the wife.

Then Mickie found out about the page I hadn't told her about. Even the on duty supervisor, the previously discussed Mack Cutter of the uncertain judgment, was angry I had led my cute blue eyed partner into danger without even warning her. He called me cowboy or John Wayne or something.

I was unrepentant. There had been cops and firemen all over the place.

"Well," I said to Mickie. "How was I to know you were going to be hugging the murderer?"

That got her even more furious.

"Promise me you will never tell anyone about that," she said.

I stopped riding with her. I was sure she was either going to kill a patient or cost a paramedic his job. But she still managed to get me into a whole lot of trouble later when I picked up a shift for someone that she happened to be on. It was again through poor judgment, insubordination and doing the wrong thing, to wit counselling a PE patient to slow his breathing down, as if he were hyper ventilating, instead of doing what I told her to do.

That's another story though.

10 HAZING

I don't know how it is in law enforcement, but in EMS there's not much hazing, compared to Fire. Too busy most of the time, and too young a service for traditions, perhaps.

Occasionally, however, it's hard to resist. I had a new Basic who was working with a patient in the back. Training someone new is called 'driving from the back' and 'patient care from the front,' if you follow. You have to solve medical problems for your partner while you're driving, and give street directions while you're in back working a patient. He had found that the patient's blood sugar was 50, that is, ten points below normal. If the patient is altered mental, that means IV access and D50 (50% glucose) IV. This patient was not feeling good, but perfectly able to swallow safely, so that meant oral glucose.

"I'll get some glucose," I said, still standing by the side door of the truck. I was assisting, thus. Oral glucose comes in a little toothpaste type tube containing a gel saturated with 15 grams of glucose. "Ask him if he likes strawberry or lime?"

The patient wanted strawberry.

Now, oral glucose only comes in one, you could call it flavor, I suppose, though I've heard it tastes as nasty as something which is almost pure sugar can taste. About as bad as nitroglycerin mixed with baby aspirin, if you can stand an in joke. (The acute cardiac oral med regimen.)

"Here you go," I said, handing up the tube. Then I went up to the front, started the truck and pulled out.

Took my new Basic a few minutes to get the tube open and figure out how to squirt the contents down the patient's throat. But soon enough I hear,

"HEY! THIS ISN'T STRAWBERRY!"

11 THE WOMAN WHO ATE HER BABY

We took a call for a psych transport out of a doctor's office in a strip mall. The office was hard to find since malls and businesses don't post their street numbers anymore. In fact, one of the tips I could give people is to hide their street numbers better if they don't want us to find them. If everyone in your neighborhood has their number posted by their garage doors, and you post yours on a tree, or you find it cute to stencil it on a rock, letting it fade with the rains, or you hang it from a tree and let the branches grow over it, we will find your house anyway. It may take us a bit longer, though, just enough time to turn a full arrest or an asthma attack or an allergic reaction into a fatality. Even if you don't post a street number at all, we can usually find you by extrapolation. Some medics have a real talent for it.

You might also consider, if you live in a gated community, whether the likelihood of getting robbed or kidnapped or burgled is greater than of having a fire or medical emergency. In theory our dispatcher will have or ask for the gate code, if that all works out right, but even so it will slow up the ambulance. The crime rate in the US is the lowest it has ever been, not just in our history but probably in human history, but people still die of trauma or disease at the same rate as always. That is, 100%. Everyone.

So we parked next to the handicapped ramp, got out our stretcher and marched in. An attendant showed us which exam room to go to. We found a 30 y/o female of mixed race with her infant, maybe two months old. I took a good look before asking for the information packet and talking to the provider. Physically, Adriana was clearly in good shape, breathing well, good color, good muscle tone, alert, moving all extremities; psychologically, she did not look or act bizarre, though her color was a bit greyish and she had some facial droop.

The doc attributed this to Bell's palsy, which was plausible, but kept stroke still in play. The doc was a small oriental woman in her 40's with a slight accent. She was practicing in a store front in a bad neighborhood. She further informed me that Adriana had a history of schizophrenia and cocaine abuse, and that she was delusional, for which the doc was transporting her to an emergency department for medical clearance in route to a psych facility. This was not an emergency detention. Adriana was going of her own free will.

I asked the doc if she had run a tox screen. A toxicology urine test for drugs. She said, no, the patient says she has not been using. I scrupulously hid my skepticism, though my partners tell me my control of body language is poor. One of them can do a good imitation of me hanging my head to one side in despair and disbelief. The fact is, no one who deals with addicts ever believes a word they say about anything.

I'm perfectly sympathetic to addicts. We all of us without exception have compulsions and obsessions and addictions, whether to tobacco, food, bad marriage choices, shopping, alcohol, the internet, you name it, and some of us are unfortunate enough to have really bad ones which wreck our lives. It's some kind of disease or disorder. But that doesn't mean I buy anything an addict says. In my experience, and everyone else's, addicts lie about things they don't even need to lie about, things that don't even do them any credit, much less about their drug use.

But I do have a great deal of respect for MDs. I have rarely run into one who wasn't kind, personable, and of course much more knowledgeable about medicine than I am. Maybe she was busy and figured the ER would just repeat the tox screen anyway.

The office had a plain, linoleum, nondescript look, was maybe less than half full of patients, with only a few people in the waiting room.

We had to wait a few minutes while Adriana finished feeding her baby. She held him on her lap with total absorption, staring into his face with look of astonished fascination. It was not normal. It kind of reminded me of a film I had once seen of an adolescent female gorilla looking at another more mature gorilla feeding her baby. Adriana was so simple we suspected some mental retardation.

We assembled our paperwork, making sure we had demographics including SS no, DOB and insurance info; a history of some kind; and a list of drugs the patient took. There was not much there. In fact, the doc had not seen her before today.

Adriana was friendly and cooperative. I never felt threatened, though at no time will I turn my back on a psych patient, and I'm cautious about passing close to them. I tell them everything I'm doing, don't stare at them but keep a little eye contact going. If they are agitated I figure out if they want to be left alone or if they would like to talk. I try to steer them away from obsession and try not to reinforce their delusions, but I also try to be as unaggressive and unthreatening as possible, while making sure not to cringe or withdraw either. Keep a solid presence. Don't back down, but also don't get yourself in a position where you are being asked to back down. You get used to psych patients. They don't scare you merely by being crazy anymore. Most of them are quite obviously not threatening at all and arouse no discomfort in the experienced provider, but quite a few of those who need emergency transport do make you nervous.

We seat-belted the baby's car seat to the captain's chair behind the stretcher, so I had to sit next to the patient on the bench. Since she was so cooperative, this was less awkward than it could have been. We checked the baby for color, tone, behavior briefly just to be sure we didn't have a second patient. You can tell a huge amount about a child just by looking. If their eye contact, breathing and skin tone are all normal, it's unlikely they are in any immediate danger. The eyes may be the window of the soul, but in small children the skin is the painting of their health status. The patient never once during transport turned around to look at her child. Again, not normal.

Adriana told me she was seeing things, and that things looked distorted. What things? The baby's face seemed to be changing.

I found that ominous too. Command voices are about the most dangerous delusions, but ones related to relatives, particularly helpless relatives, are not good either.

Still, transport was uneventful. This was not a call where we had to struggle with the patient or keep them quiet or sedate them or restrain them. Still, I did not like this picture at all, so I copiously documented everything. I reported to the receiving nurse at the emergency room that no tox screen had been run and that Adriana had a history of drug abuse, that the facial droop might not be Bell's palsy, but someone should consider stroke. A stroke is usually slurred speech or one-sided paralysis, but it can be vision changes or confusion or in fact anything, since we are talking about the brain.

And then of course there was schizophrenic decompensation, which was differential number one. But the last. A diagnosis of exclusion, since there is no blood test or scan for it. Not that it's hard to diagnose once you rule out sepsis, low blood sugar and the like. And it's also clearly a medical problem. Schizophrenics don't even look right, much less act right.

So at destination we cleared without further incident, but I can tell you what happened next in detail. I talked to the SAFD medic who took her next call, I read the newspaper, and I took a phone call from the private detective assigned to her legal case. I also heard from the nursing staff at the ER where we took her.

Adriana had been released to her family after a few tests had been run. Never admitted to a psych ward. She lived next door to her sister, so someone figured the sister could keep track of her. This is not a good hospital by the way. Adriana denied wanting to hurt herself or anyone else.

Well, we err on the side of personal freedom in this country, rather than on the side of protecting people from themselves. If someone wants to kill themselves or someone else, basically, they can. Unless some really clever provider figures out that's what the patient's plan is and figures out some way to commit her.

We once had an ex-marine who owned a rifle who I thought was intent on killing herself. I told the doc. He more or less shrugged. If she really wants to do it and she's determined, she will. He was busy with patients he could help.

We knew a guy who liked to ride his mobile wheelchair on rural roads around his house at night. My partner said he should be taken off the streets. I pointed out that it was not against the law to be stupid. As long as he knew who he was, where he was and what the date was, he could do what he wanted. Ride a motorcycle, own a gun, whatever.

The worst though was they released the infant with Adriana. I would like to hear the excuse for that one. I know Child Protective Services is over-worked, but really.

Things went OK for a day or two, or at least no one called 911. Then the sister did.

The crew entered the house to find Adriana wailing "I killed my baby."

In fact, she had skinned it, opened the skull and eaten part of the brains. The infant was unsalvageable and Adriana was brought by police to wherever they hold the criminally insane while they determine what to do. I next saw her name in the newspaper.

So did my boss and supervisor. They pulled my run-form and were pleased to see all the documentation. At least the ambulance company hadn't missed a trick. The original doc had pretty much done the right things too.

The PI called me for info to help her lawyer. The first time he called I told him I couldn't really tell him anything without a release from either the patient or a court. The second time he pretended he had filed this documentation at my HQ. I do not believe what journalists or PIs tell me any more than addicts, but, in the first place, I wanted to get this information off my chest, and, in the second, I wanted to be as much help as possible to this patient in getting her the right treatment and adjudication. Nothing I was going to say was detrimental to her. So I told him most of the above.

Months later I read she had been judged insane and admitted for treatment to some city facility. Mental health care is poor in my state, but at least she wasn't in prison, where most of our mentally ill get their treatment, such as it is.

The week the news came out, though, I happened to be on the floor of another hospital, picking up another patient, when I heard the nurses at the nurses' station discussing the case. I told them I had transported her. This is legal public information.

One of them said, "Well, I think she should get the death penalty." An RN who doesn't believe that diseases cause aberrant behavior. I wondered if she thought her septic patients were faking it too.

I looked her over. Dyed blond hair, fake nails, overweight. No doubt a religious conservative, but surely not one who appreciated the appearance God had given her.

I said, "She skinned her baby, opened the skull and ate its brains. .What, exactly, would she have to do to convince you that she was crazy?"

12 THE MORE COMPLAINTS, THE BETTER

Medics soon realize that the more complaints a patient has, the less worried you have to be. If an obese guy with a history of heart problems tells you he feels pressure in his chest, you need to be extremely concerned about him, even if his EKG comes out normal. This sounds like an MI. If a woman tells you she just got a really bad headache, unlike any she ever had before, same. Cerebral aneurysm comes to mind.

But if someone tells you their head hurts, their chest hurts, their stomach hurts, everything hurts, and they're nauseous and have been throwing up, and they feel terrible, that's unlikely to be anything, except maybe flu. If they have pain on palpation in a particular area, there's likely to be something really wrong there. If they hurt everywhere you touch them, that's more likely to be chronic pain syndrome or fibromyalgia. Medical conditions, maybe, but not at all emergent.

Nausea and vomiting feel terrible. Make you wish you were dead. But these complaints are rarely an emergency. If abdominal pain comes on suddenly and is accompanied by blood pressure drop, radiation to the back, and a throbbing mass in the abdomen, that could be an abdominal aortic aneurysm. Triple A. If it's lower right quadrant and has gotten worse and worse, it could be appendicitis. 99% of the time, though, Abominable Pain is non emergent. N/V/D, nausea/vomiting/diarrhea, is not an alarming presentation.

Don't get me wrong. Abominable pain and n/v/d can be symptoms of many serious conditions, even fatal ones, like cancer, bowel obstructions and the like, but except for the triple A, maybe the appy, these are not hot transports. These patients may die--but not in your truck, they won't. Whereas the wheezy asthmatic or the older guy with the unexplained dizzy spell or the droopy mouth may.

Less is more.

13 TRANSPORTED

My first EMS book, *Earn Money Sleeping*, was about 911 calls. This one is mostly about the transport service I worked for later. On the average, medics work 911 for about 5 to 8 years. 24 hours on, 48 off, 365 days a year. Maybe a two week vacation. After that, most go on to other things. At my transport ambulance service, I work 9 to 9, MWF, for better pay. I started at 4 days a week, but even then it was much less stressful. Probably half of all medics working are working for transport services, and every medic has done transports, often for his 911 service.

We service nursing homes, medical facilities, dialysis clinics, doctor's offices, wound care facilities, private individuals who need ambulance transport, some of whom do not trust the local 911 service, or have been turned down for emergent transport, and the like.

All these people call us for routine transports, but also for emergencies.

Still, these calls tend to be less dramatic. You rarely get to enter someone's home, figure out what his problem is yourself, and take your own initiative to deal with it. You intubate rarely, do fewer full cardiac arrests. You tend to have more elderly patients. Your trauma will be falls in nursing homes rather than motor vehicle or farm accidents.

Still, you do just as many IV's, and you actually deal with medical problems more frequently, since your client population is so frail and ill. It's good training for beginning medics. They get to hear a lot of bad lungs in a short time, see a lot of sick people, and, if they are conscientious, check out a lot of drug regimens and histories. But even for experienced medics-- actually, especially for experienced medics-- medical calls are ultimately more interesting than trauma. Major trauma is dramatic but, besides being rare, it's also all the same. Stop the bleeding, rarely other interventions, backboard, C-collar, transport, IV in route, call it in. Don't get me wrong, it's fun. More often, though, you will get fender benders, or even totaled, smashed vehicles, with patients who just complain of some neck pain, and, by the time they get to the ED, have a major complaint of backboard pain. Which you communicate to the MD to let him know he can stand down.

The medical calls tend to be more complex. Is a breathing problem lung related or cardiac?

You have to decide what to do about it without x ray or diagnostic equipment. If a patient is unconscious, or altered mental, why is he unconscious? What should you do about it?

Furthermore, your transport patients are almost always really sick and really need an ambulance, unlike most 911 callers. 85% of 911 patients do not need emergent transport to an emergency room. Well over half don't need an ambulance at all. Family disturbances in the middle of the night (assault), fender-benders, flu, minor fractures, false alarms, people who call 911 because their car isn't working.

You get called by a home health nurse because her patient is cyanotic. You arrive to find, instead of a Smurf, the patient walking and talking. You look at the home health attendant. She points to a blue spot under the side of the patient's ankle. Kind of like the one under my own boot. You transport.

So transport calls will often be less dramatic, mostly, but frequently quite interesting. It's a world apart. Some new skills are required too: using IV pumps, Bi-Pap machines and mechanical vents. All of which can and do go wrong.

There's always a delicate balance to maintain, too, because most transport patients have been triaged by a medical professional before you arrive, whether it's a physician in an ER or his office, or an LVN in a nursing home. Not infrequently, some of them are professional in name only, and have completely misunderstood or mismanaged a patient. So you have to intervene without offending the LVN. Or nursing home director, whose chief qualification for her job, as far as I can tell, is being able to wear copious amounts of make-up and navigate high heels without them improving her mood or character at all. Experienced in sales, I think. But still your superior.

Couple examples, and how I learned the skills to deal with them. Or not. Maybe not my most exciting chapter.

This nursing home turned out to be notorious, had I known. We'll call it Field and Stream so I don't get sued. It didn't look that bad, no pervasive smell of old urine, but, just as an example, a week or so later, I took a patient from there to the ED. She had already been diagnosed by an MD as a UTI (urinary tract infection), and prescribed medication, but then they transported her anyway.

When I gave report to the ER nurse, she was working with a trainee, who said, "I don't understand why they transported. Why not wait to see if the antibiotics work?"

"Oh, I can explain that in three words," said the regular RN.

"What?"

"Field and Stream."

Anyway, earlier, before we were wised up, we got called for a psych transport from this place. It's in an outlying town. We were asked to take a resident to a distant hospital with a psych floor, to be evaluated by their ER before being admitted to psych. The nursing home is a pleasant looking, brick place set in soothing countryside. Which shows looks can be deceiving.

The patient was an elderly, slender Jewish lady--kind of urban for the unsophisticated setting--accompanied by her sister, who, unlike our patient, was compos mentis, though pretty slow on her mental feet. Both in their 80's.

She was going for "psych," not otherwise specified. I looked over her chart, saw she had a history of psychosis, dementia and diabetes. Three nurses were far too busy chatting at the nursing station to talk to us. Actually, not even chatting, which might have been over their skill level. Kind of vegetating or staring blankly into space. Wiping drool off their faces from time to time.

Since I was taking the patient via the ER, not directly to the psych floor, I did have to give report in route.

"What kind of symptoms has she been having?"

"She's already been examined by a medical professional."

"Yeah, but I do have to give report and write it up."

"Psych symptoms."

"Like what?" I'm shortening this in order to relieve the boredom somewhat. It was like pulling teeth. They were yawning infectiously.

"Well, she's been combative," they finally allowed.

She weighed all of 90 pounds.

"How is that different from her baseline? It says here she's got a history of psychosis." Now I know that when people don't know the answers to questions they are supposed to know the answers to, they can get hostile and defensive. These questions seemed really simple though.

"She's already been examined by a medical professional." (Just drive the fucking ambulance, asshole!)

A medical professional?! Chiropractor? Phlebotomist? LVN? Why not say doctor, if that's what you mean? Surely not the director of nursing!

Just to give you the back story here, they seemed to feel that, as the patient had already been evaluated, my only job was just to get her to where their MD, or whoever it was, had decided she needed to go, and not waste their time. However, the way ambulance transports to emergency rooms work, is that the medic must call the patient in to the ER in route, and, at a minimum, give age, sex, vitals, chief complaint, ETA and any relevant findings or interventions, as well as answer the receiving MD or RN's questions sensibly. Then, when we get to the ER, we give a second more comprehensive report to the MD or RN, usually MD if the patient is emergent.

Then, too, if a patient is sick enough to require an ambulance, there is every likelihood that she will either require some intervention in route, or need to be upgraded to emergent if she crashes, and then re-routed to the nearest appropriate facility. In order to do this effectively, a medic needs to know the patient's complaints, history, medications and what has already been done or discovered.

Now, if I were really suave, I would have been able to explain all this to the LVNs without offending them, as they seemed not to know any of the normal procedures for sending a patient via ambulance from a nursing home to an emergency room. However, this would have been really tricky to do. It would be a little like going into a bakery and explaining to the baker that he needed to knead the dough, and then put it in the oven, before selling it. It's hard to believe, though, that a baker would just hand you a pile of...uh, unbaked dough. Or that he would take kindly to being instructed how to bake bread. It frankly never occurred to me this could be ignorance. Nursing homes send patients to emergency rooms on a daily basis. Several times a day would not be unusual. A lay reader may, hopefully, be interested in how that all works, but a nursing home LVN could hardly escape having it explained to her on her first day, or preferably, before she was hired.

Anyway, I gave this line of questioning up. Not getting anywhere. We were in the patient's room by this time, with her sister listening.

"What was her D stick?" I asked the nurse. Her blood sugar. I could have taken it myself, but my boss doesn't like for us to bring too much equipment into the nursing home, as previous LVN's complained we were doing unnecessary diagnostics, thinking we were doing it to charge more. We don't charge more. And I do have to report a D stick on every medical patient to the ER, I told my boss. They ask. Otherwise we look bad there. Especially with a patient exhibiting altered mentation. Do it on the truck, my boss instructed.

The LVN flounced off.

One strong likelihood here was that the patient's blood sugar was too low, causing her psych symptoms. Possibly she had taken her insulin but not eaten enough. Very common.

Nurse flounces back in. Grabs patient by back of arm without saying anything to her, stabs her with the lancet to obtain blood for the accucheck. Patient leaps and squirms. Combative, you see.

Nurse flounces out.

The sister says, "Well, what was it"?

"Oh, it only says HI," LVN says. Leaves.

HI on an accucheck means over 400, or over 600, depending on the instrument. Four to six times normal blood sugar. Morbid. The opposite of what I had conjectured. Given all the care diabetics normally get nowadays, you usually see low blood sugars, caused by taking too much insulin, or taking insulin and not eating, or taking insulin while nausea and vomiting are depleting nutrition. Not so much the old classical high blood sugars of untreated diabetes. Like this patient.

Diabetes means insulin is not moving enough sugar from the blood to storage, so untreated diabetics have high blood sugars. The sugar is necrotic. Destroys things. Vessels, kidneys, brain. So diabetics check their blood sugars, take medicines like insulin, and control their diets to avoid this. The compliant ones.

So this patient had eaten. Staff had just neglected to give her insulin. For days, probably. And never checked her blood sugar.

So my choices at this point were (A) transport this patient emergent to the nearest appropriate facility, which is protocol for a blood sugar over 400 and altered mental status. Or (B) get the staff to give her insulin. We don't carry insulin on board. Not an emergency intervention.

(A) would mightily piss everyone off, as arrangements had already been made, hopefully in consult with an MD, to take her to the distant hospital. And, other than by EMS protocol, it didn't seem really necessary. The patient had been altered mental for a while, and medically was pretty stable, good vitals, color, etc.

So we asked the nurse. She did the flounce again. Left. Surprisingly, though, she did come back by the time we had the patient on the stretcher ready to go. Injected insulin. Flounced off.

My partner, who has even less patience for this kind of stuff than I do, set out for the nurses' station. Namely, we had to know how much insulin she had given. When he got there, he told me, the three nurses were gossiping about me. They didn't like me. Brash was the word they used.

"How much insulin did you give her?" he said, shortly. Then he wheeled around and came back.

The nursing home director shows up.

"Is there a problem?" she asks. "Are you ready to transport yet?" She's polite, but markedly not pleased to have been involved at all. At least she looks like a reasonable person, which is something.

"No problem," we say. "We're transporting right now." We could have stopped everything to tell the whole story to her to try to clear up the misunderstanding, obviously created by the LVNs' complaints, but delaying transport to get into a "he said, she said" didn't seem to me something I wanted to do. She hired those nurses and retained them. Though, it must be said, nursing homes are chronically understaffed, and they are not the plum job in the nursing world. The cream of the crop go into ICU or ER. Or specialties like OB GYN or PICU. So even if I push my very sick patient's stretcher up against the wall and spend whatever time the director has patience for trying to, in effect, reform her notorious nursing home, it's doubtful I would get anywhere. Many nursing home directors don't even seem to know any medicine, particularly not those in charge of independent living or assisted living facilities. In this case, this being a specialized nursing facility (SNF, sniff), she should know her medicine, but if so, how did her facility get the reputation it has?

Instead we transport.

So then she calls my boss to complain. I hear from the latter that they have been friends, or at least acquaintances, for years. My boss appears either not to know anything about the reputation of this place or not to care. "How is berating them going to help?" She is pissed at us. From her point of view, it doesn't matter what the problem was. She wants the nursing home to call her for all their transports. Period.

Long explanations to her have to be used sparingly. Like maybe once every ten years. She has other things to do, and verbiage just seems to affix the incident more firmly in her mind. Under the file name "medic fucking up."

I took the patient to her distant hospital. She was following a little dog around the ambulance with her eyes, and complaining about the way we were dealing with it--in a nice way, though. We don't stock small dogs in the ambulance, actually. Sweet lady.

The ER doc didn't seem that interested in her blood sugar either. So we just thanked her politely and left. Nothing else to do, and the likelihood of an ER doc not knowing how to handle a case like this is slim. Maybe the nursing home had called and warned her about us.

Another time I'm running emergent practically from headquarters, having just come on shift, to another nursing home, for a patient with heart problems. I trot in to an exquisitely over-decorated, huge reception area. My patient is sitting on a bench, looking at me alertly. Across from her is a woman on the phone, the receptionist. The patient is elderly and appears reasonably healthy, but she does have some dementia, and is not telling me much. I ask the receptionist what the problem is. She holds up her hand. I'm rudely interrupting her important conversation on the phone, apparently. To my overhearing, it doesn't seem to me to equal an emergency heart problem.

Turns out she doesn't know any more than the demented patient. Doesn't seem to be a lot sharper either. Has no documentation. I ask her to get me some assistance, at least our info packet. She hasn't gotten over my uncouth entry.

The director of the facility floats slowly into view, like a great white circling prey.

She's made up and dressed to kill. Barely recognizable as a human being. Had I recognized that she considered herself to be an august personage, things would have gone better, but I was distracted by assessing a patient with an emergency heart problem, supposedly. The Director is mightily exercised by having to condescend to telling an emergency crew about her resident. She does allow that the patient is probably in atrial fibrillation, since she has had that before. She does not seem to know what a fib is, though. "Well, she's assisted living, so we don't have medical records." All they have is her meds, which they dole out to her per prescription. It may seem bizarre to you that her caretakers don't know what the meds are for, but there it is.

"It would be useful if you knew her history. What was the outcome last time she had this? Do you know what was done for her?" Nope, not in her job description. Which is selling the place to sons and daughters of prospective residents. You'd think she could better assist them in living if she knew something about their medical history, which is why they are in assisted living in the first place. But I was new at transports. The world of elder care was still new territory.

We were both, me and the director, astounded. She had never even contemplated being rousted out of her luxurious office by a mere ambulance driver to answer questions about one of her residents, much less having the uniformed flunky "answer back" when she chunked shit at him from her high horse. I mean, she had not risen to her present heights in order to be addressed as an equal by some low level uniformed personnel.

Meanwhile, being new to transport service, and coming from 911 work, I was used to focusing a 100% on the patient's welfare, and having everyone assist me, including several firemen, law enforcement officers, passersby, family, what have you. Now, running into uncooperative family members, bystanders or neighbors is nothing new, but the remedy had always been simple. You ignore them, or if they are really in your way, you remove them from the scene, if necessary in cuffs belonging to a sheriff's officer.

Astounded? Perhaps appalled is the right word.

The answers I did get were curt. Grudging is putting it too mildly.

"Why are you being rude?" I said finally.

"Well, in the first place, you took 30 minutes to respond to this emergency call."

"Not my fault. What was the second thing?"

"Excuse me?!"

She thought I was being smart, but I was sincerely responding to her list. Turns out the way to handle this is to say, "I'm sorry, please call the number on this card to find out what happened. My crew responded immediately," but I just gave up and turned away to give full attention to my patient, who I had been simultaneously evaluating anyway.

In other words, none of this would have happened if 1. I had been more experienced. 2. We had not been or perceived to be slow to respond, and 3. had not most of my attention been taken up with assessing the patient, or if 4. she had really been in bad shape. Then I would have been hustling her out of there, documents, history or not, and instantly dropped any queries which didn't bear immediate fruit or slowed me down. It was kind of a perfect storm scenario. Though not untypical of transport work.

The patient was in a fib, and RVR (rapid ventricular response), which means the atrium of her heart, the upper chamber, was fibrillating, instead of beating in a normal, orderly way. A fib in itself not a dangerous arrhythmia, unlike ventricular fibrillation, but, in addition to that, her heart ventricles (lower chambers) were responding to the fibrillation by beating too fast, which could be dangerous for her blood pressure, mental status, perfusion and the like. Though she seemed to be tolerating it well enough. After years of experience I have learned that some of these nursing home patients are more or less continuously in a fib and have adapted to it quite well. Requires transport and careful monitoring, but it's not the emergency presented by a person at home who suddenly develops the rhythm, feels terrible, calls you and really has compromised vitals. Whose heart is beating too fast to fill and pump good volume.

Atrial fibrillation can even be found in a healthy young person who has overindulged. It's then called holiday heart. The main danger is that the fibrillations can throw blood clots. Whereas ventricular fibrillation is immediately lethal. The atrial kick is less than 10% of the heart's ejection fraction: output. The ventricle is the true pump.

If a patient in a fib is severely symptomatic, you can cardiovert. 100 joules shock.

It doesn't work. The heart stops, patient goes unconscious (this is alarming), then the heart starts up again with some normal beats, and pretty soon, a fib again. They do cardiovert in hospitals, though, and cardioversion is in our protocols, so it must work sometimes. It never has for me. I've successfully shocked several kinds of bad rhythms, but a fib is really stubborn.

The reason you only do it when the patient is severely symptomatic is that the shock can throw clots too. Normally the patient is put on blood thinners for a while before cardioversion. Of course, a lot of a fib patients are already on blood thinners.

Another thing you can do is administer a calcium channel blocker, IV. It keeps the heart from beating too fast. However, since you can only give it to patients with a systolic BP over 120, as it can cause hypotension, it's not very useful either. Because most severely symptomatic patients are having blood pressure problems already.

This lady was not severely symptomatic. No chest pain, no hypotension. She was altered mental in the sense that she was a poor historian, but this appeared to be a stable chronic condition rather than caused by her arrhythmia. That is, she was alert and perky, she did not look really sick, she was not lethargic or dizzy or...it's hard to describe. There's a difference between an Alzheimer's patient, and one who is not getting adequate perfusion to her brain. Or has a head injury. Not enough difference to let your guard down, or for a medical diagnosis, but enough for a working field impression.

Technically, medics don't "diagnose." But if you don't figure out what's wrong, and do something appropriate about it, you're not doing your job.

Nevertheless, I did run her hot to the hospital, getting an IV in route, in case her condition did deteriorate. Now I might not. Elderly nursing home residents do get different care than patients in other demographics. It may seem invidious not to treat everyone equally, and it can be. You can fail to recognize that a woman is having a heart attack because pre-menopausal women hardly ever have them. But you can also recognize that she IS having a heart attack because you realize that her atypical symptoms, like fainting or dizziness or back pain, can indicate a heart attack in someone in that demographic.

So the director was so pissed she cancelled the contract with our service. She kept muttering, my boss told me, about "that old man" (me). I hadn't said anything which to my mind was rude, but one skill these sales people do have is reading body language and unspoken sentiments. In this case, unalloyed contempt.

My boss did not even want to hear my side, basically. She had lost a contract, the greatest sin a medic could encompass. She also found out that we had responded in a timely way. The delay had been at the nursing home end. So to her mind that meant "response time was not an issue." Well, maybe not to her, but that's what set the nursing home director off to start with.

I think that was the closest I got to being fired at this service. To give her her due, my boss was always ready to give someone a second chance, if she thought their attitude was worth working with.

Well, this was all quite a change from 911. Where, if someone gets in the way of your patient care, you have them removed from the scene, by law enforcement in handcuffs if necessary, and you are always accompanied by at least 2 and as many as 6 firemen and cops, who all understand your perspective quite well, and have no more than professional patience for 'citizens.' Obstructing a public servant is a felony. At an MVA scene, cops won't even let anyone to get close enough to you for it to happen.

So there are a lot of medics who can't stand this kind of work and consider it beneath their dignity. They stay in 911 or go into fire or get their RN or leave the profession. Still, with a few basic stratagems, you can maintain friendly relations with staff, and the patients themselves can be rewarding. It's always more fun to get along with people than not, unless you have some serious anger management issues, which in some cases might be truly justified. Anger at injustice has its uses. But most medical staff are nice people. They go into a helping profession for good reasons. And like all workplaces, theirs can be pretty boring, so an entertaining medic with some friendly repartee can be enjoyed by all. Most of the staff you deal with are competent, nice, cheerful people who enjoy their work. Which is more than you can say about most professions, I think. Even many of the staffers who are historically lacking in good study habits and clinical insight, to put it politely, are generally compassionate and at least trying to do a good job. There are however enough exceptions to guarantee that you will have to deal with a less estimable person at least once a week of not oftener. And deal with them in a different way than if you are on a 911 crew. So these may not be the most enticing stories to introduce EMS. They do give you an idea of what life on the other side is like, though. Otherwise, check out *Earn Money Sleeping*.

And there is no strategy which will help you get along with everyone, all the same. You have to consider that 1 out of 10 people has a psychotic episode some time in their life, and it could be just at the moment you're asking them if their patient is diabetic. Maybe they are interpreting your question as obscene remarks about their mother.

Just don't let the despair show.

If you're really good, you could develop the acting ability to indicate, by your facial expression, that you consider a given LVN to be an outstanding professional, even though she has failed to take the blood sugar of her altered mental patient, who is diabetic, even after having been clued in that there might be something wrong there, by the fact that the patient hasn't gotten her insulin for days. I never did develop that. But I can do the 'I'm just the ambulance driver, give me whatever paperwork you can spare and tell me where to go' look.

To be honest, on scene I don't really have the mental capacity to judge staff the way I will afterwards when thinking it over. At the time, all I'm doing is pushing to get what I need for the patient. I compensate for having a small motor upstairs by having a really good transmission, so I can focus all its minimal power where most needed. Think of me as a Porsche.

Then again, I have been diagnosed with OBS. Obnoxious Personality Disorder. I'd go to our support group meetings, but we can't stand each other. I do plan to get a handicapped sticker though. Workman's Comp.

So I hope you enjoy these stories even if they are not as exciting as 911 calls. Even in my 911 book, I was more focused on what the profession is like, seen from the inside, what you might call the human dimension, than physical drama. It's there, all right, but it's not fires and gunshots. The aftermath of fires and gunshots, saving the victims, can be equally urgent and dramatic, but not as visual. Takes place in close quarters, not the wide screen, and requires some thought.

14 MR. HUTCHINS

We were dropping off a patient at a middling good nursing home when we passed an elderly gentleman sitting in the hallway in a wheelchair, earnestly puzzling over a document.

"Could you please help me?" he asked plaintively. He was a very pleasant looking, well groomed and nicely dressed fellow, wearing pressed chinos and a nice clean men's shirt with a subtle check pattern. He had something about him which suggested some distinction. We were pushing the stretcher at the time, so I said, "I'll be back in minute. Let me get this stretcher squared away."

Normally, that might be the end of it. An elderly patient in a nursing home might not even remember what he needed by the time you got back to him, and it's staff's job to take care of their patients. We have ours to deal with. We've been in paint-peeling and verminous hell houses which stank of old infected urine, had a gaggle of drooling inmates slumped over in wheelchairs around the nursing station, and whose sound track consisted of the ceaseless monotonous cries of a woman calling "Help me, help me" in a voice which would have aroused despair in a demon.

This call was my partner's, though, so I had nothing to do while he dealt with the paperwork and gave report. Besides, something struck me about Mr. Hutchins, as his name turned out to be. Plus, I was probably in the right mood, perhaps.

So I when I passed by his room with the stretcher, I stopped, and he handed me the paper, which he was still looking at anxiously.

It was a piece of some medical document, a fragment.

Mr. Hutchins looked up at me.

"Oh, you don't have to worry about this, sir," I said. "Staff will take care of it. It's not a problem at all."

Mr. Hutchins looked very relieved. He thanked me politely.

I started to talk to him.

"Do you have family coming here to visit you?"

"I think so," he said, puzzled.

Turns out he did not know where he was, how he had got there, or who was taking care of him. Naturally this made him anxious, but he took it very bravely, I thought. What he did know was what he had done for a living before. He was an engineer.

It happened we got to that nursing home quite a bit in subsequent shifts. I got in the habit of stopping by to talk to Mr. Hutchins. My regular partner at that time got to be fond of him too.

Mr. Hutchins could remember pretty much every detail of engineering jobs he had done 40 and 50 years ago, many of them in South America, where he had built bridges. He was always pleasant and well groomed.

Oddly enough, he recognized us every time. But he still couldn't recall if he had family living nearby or what city he was in now, even though he remembered Bogota quite well.

Then one day he was gone. He seemed to be in quite good health, so while it's possible he had a crisis and was taken to a hospital, it's more likely his family moved him to another location. I hope it was home. He clearly couldn't live by himself, but he also wasn't a lot of trouble to take care of, being cooperative, able to move himself around, eat his own meals and so on. Still, if everyone is working long hours, the way people do nowadays, they can't be around the house to look after him.

One Hispanic gentleman we dealt with had been taking care of his mother just fine at home, until he realized she could not stay at his house alone any more while he was at work. He moved her to a nursing home, where she fell and broke her hip. Basically, this killed her. She was too old to recuperate from a broken hip, cooperate with rehab, so she was bedbound. People usually don't last long bedbound. Mammals gotta move. Can't lie there motionless for a month like a croc or a snake. And nursing homes can't prevent people from falling, unless they figure out how to adapt one of those baby walker things for old people. Tying them to the bed, or jailing them within bedrails, besides being cruel, is making them bedbound even before they need to be.

We couldn't ask staff about Mr. Hutchins. Since he wasn't our patient, all the information the nursing staff had about him was privileged, under the HIPAA laws which protect patient's privacy.

Unreadable Traffic

Short term memory goes first. Mine isn't what it used to be either.

www.ingramcontent.com/pod-product-compliance
Lightning Source LLC
Chambersburg PA
CBHW051806170526
45167CB00005B/1900